Orthodontic Treatment Mechanics and the Preadjusted Appliance

Orthodontic Treatment Mechanics and the Preadjusted Appliance

John C. Bennett *LDS, DOrth*
London, UK

Richard P. McLaughlin *DDS*
San Diego, California
USA

Wolfe Publishing

Copyright © 1993 Wolfe Publishing, an imprint of Mosby–Year
Book Europe Ltd
Printed by BPCC Hazells Ltd, Aylesbury, England
ISBN 0 7234 1906X

A CIP catalogue record for this book is available from the British
Library.

For full details of all Mosby–Year Book Europe Ltd titles please write
to Mosby–Year Book Europe Ltd, Brook House, 2–16 Torrington
Place, London WC1E 7LT, England.

Contents

Preface

There have been numerous changes in orthodontics over the past 30 years, which have profoundly affected the profession. These include the introduction of direct bonding agents and more effective cementing materials, the use of ceramic and sapphire brackets, and the development of more efficient and effective archwires, to name only a few. However, none of these changes has had a more profound effect on the profession than the introduction of the preadjusted appliance system.

Prior to the 1970s, there were minor appliance adjustments made in the direction of preadjusted appliances (i.e. tipping of the brackets to minimize the need for second order bends), but it was not until Lawrence F. Andrews' evaluation and measurement of the non-orthodontic normal study models, followed by his development of the Andrews Straight-Wire® Appliance, that the preadjusted appliance became a sophisticated three-dimensional system commercially available to the orthodontist. The introduction of this appliance affected orthodontics in two ways. First, it minimized the need for orthodontists to treat both an inadequate appliance and the dentition relative to individual tooth positioning and arch alignment. Second, it presented the possibility for a significant change in treatment mechanics, and it is this change that is the primary focus of this book, and dealt with in detail in Chapter 2.

At the outset, the authors would like to state what they wish to accomplish with this text. Orthodontic treatment can be divided into intra-arch and inter-arch considerations.

Intra-arch considerations include all manoeuvres involved in alignment and maintenance of the dentition in each individual arch. They therefore include such factors as bracket placement, archwire placement and removal, the placement of force systems within each arch, as well as miscellaneous factors such as impression taking, oral hygiene management, cavity detection, and detection of loose bands, etc.

Inter-arch considerations involve the far more difficult challenge of placing the upper and lower dentitions in three planes of space within the facial complex so that they are esthetic, fit properly during static centric occlusion, function from this static position without interferences during lateral and protrusive movements, and allow the condyles to be seated into a centric relation position within the glenoid fossae. Thus, inter-arch considerations include such factors as growth and development, and management of vertical, horizontal, and lateral skeletal and dental patterns.

The primary purpose of this text is to discuss intra-arch rather than inter-arch considerations. Within the text, there is discussion on various aspects of the preadjusted appliance system and placement of the appliance. It also includes a discussion of the six stages of orthodontic treatment, which primarily involve intra-arch considerations. The chapter on overjet reduction introduces the concept of inter-arch treatment, but the coverage of this topic is brief and is not intended to serve as a comprehensive discussion on this complex and challenging subject. In summary, it is the primary intention of the authors to present an efficient and effective way of managing intra-arch mechanics. This, in turn, will allow orthodontists to focus on inter-arch considerations.

Both extraction and non-extraction treatment are discussed in this text. However, there is an emphasis on extraction treatment, since the mechanics of these cases are generally more complex. This is not to infer that the authors treat more cases on an extraction basis than on a non-extraction basis. In fact, an attempt is made to treat without extractions whenever possible, and the authors treat a much higher percentage of cases in this manner.

This text does not provide a comparison between preadjusted orthodontic appliance systems. Since moving from the standard edgewise appliance to the preadjusted appliance, the authors have used only the Andrews Straight-Wire® Appliance. Therefore, there will be no attempt to make comparisons between this appliance and other preadjusted appliance systems. However, it is appropriate to point out that the Straight-Wire® Appliance, unlike other preadjusted appliances, was developed on a sound scientific basis, that of the non-orthodontic normal measurements made by Andrews in the early 1970s. Andrews then determined that in order to accurately transfer his non-orthodontic normal measurements to an orthodontic appliance, it was necessary to build torque into the base, rather than putting torque into the face, of the brackets. He also observed that it was also necessary to build compound contours into the base of the brackets, and that these two features allowed for level slot line-up with the appliance. These features are absent in most preadjusted appliance systems, and hence their accuracy must be questioned. The authors have found that in the treatment of numerous orthodontic cases over a 15- year period, the Straight-Wire® Appliance delivers what it claims to deliver in terms of intra-arch alignment.

Finally, the authors wish to express their thanks to two individuals for their support and guidance over the years. First, they wish to thank Lawrence F. Andrews for his effort in the development of the Straight-Wire® Appliance. They also wish to thank him for his clinical guidance over the years. Second, the authors wish to thank Maurice Berman for his contribution in the development of the six stages of orthodontic treatment relative to the preadjusted appliance system. Dr Berman worked hand-in-hand with the authors for the first six years of development of the concept and without his help and guidance, this textbook would not have come about.

Acknowledgements

The authors wish to express their thanks to the following people who have contributed to the production of this book: Susan Howes for the word-processing and preparation; John Molenaar, Dr Maurice Berman and Moira Brown for many of the line drawings and diagrams; Dr Hugo Trevisi of Presidente Prudente, Brazil, for his insights and helpful comments concerning space closure; Samuels, Rudge and Mair for the graphs in Chapter 10.

Thanks are also due to our desk editor, Jonathan Lewis, and to the editor of the *Journal of Clinical Orthodontics* for his permission to publish certain texts and diagrams which were previously published by the Journal.

1. INTRODUCTION

Historical Background

Until the mid-1970s most fixed appliance therapy was carried out using the standard edgewise bracket, either in single or twin form, having a 90° bracket base and bracket slot angulations. Archwire bending by the orthodontist was required in order to achieve adequate results.

Two major disadvantages resulted from this treatment method:

- Archwire bends were time-consuming and tedious. Even in the hands of experienced operators adjustments were imprecise and hard work, requiring hours of additional chairside attention.
- The shortcomings of the bracket system, and the extreme skill required of the orthodontist, resulted in many undertreated cases. This led to the second disadvantage. The results often appeared 'artificial'. Molars were not in a true Class I relationship, and upper incisors lacked torque. In effect, the resulting occlusion had the appearance of a 'nice orthodontic result' rather than a pleasing natural dentition. Equally important, the long-term stability of tooth alignment was compromised by failing to establish ideal tooth relationships.

Other techniques were developed and introduced into the orthodontic office. For example, the Begg approach, originating in Adelaide, Australia, was widely used in the 1960s and 1970s. It exhibited similar disadvantages to the standard edgewise method. Extensive wire bending was involved, and lack of detail control in the bracket system was reflected in the quality of results achieved by all but the most expert operators.

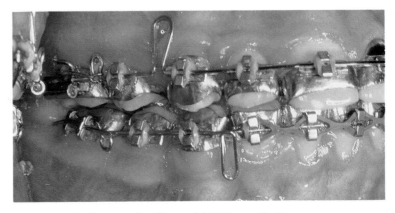

1 Standard edgewise brackets with 90° angulations.

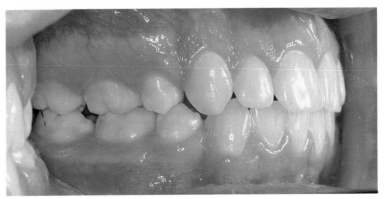

2 A typical standard edgewise type of result, between 10 and 20% undertreated in terms of molar relationship and incisor torque.

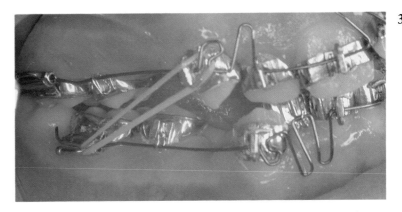

3 An early stage of a Begg treatment, showing the amount of wire bending required.

The Straight-Wire® Appliance: The Early Days

Against this background, Dr Lawrence F. Andrews developed the Straight-Wire® Appliance, which became widely available in the mid-1970s. It was hailed by clinicians as a radical step forward, offering the dual advantage of less wire bending, coupled with an improved quality of finished cases. For the first time a system seemed to offer an escape from the drudgery of wire bending. If the finishing stage of treatment was less taxing on the patient and orthodontist, then perhaps the quality of the completed case would be greatly enhanced. This would bring to a close the era of completed cases which were traditionally left 20% undertreated.

The early results with the Straight-Wire® Appliance were disappointing and much criticism was voiced. Clinicians had failed to realize that a bracket system *per se* does not offer a treatment modality. The brackets and tubes are no more than sophisticated handles, a method of attachment onto the labial surface of teeth, and thus controlling a force delivered to that surface. The force itself was generated by archwires and elastics, and it was here, in the area of treatment mechanics, that problems originated.

The old mechanics and heavy force levels, developed for standard edgewise brackets, simply did not transfer to the new, sophisticated bracket systems. Operators found that many unwanted changes occurred early in treatment in response to the heavy forces. In particular, a 'roller coaster' effect was frequently observed, with rapid, undesirable deepening of the overbite.

Another frequent observation was in the area of the premolars and canines which tended to tip and rotate into the extraction sites. Such unwanted tooth movement retarded treatment to such a great extent that the theoretical advantage offered by the new system was dramatically compromised.

4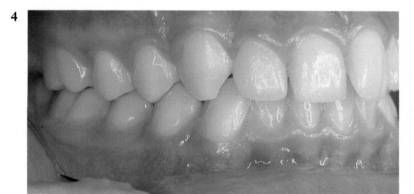
5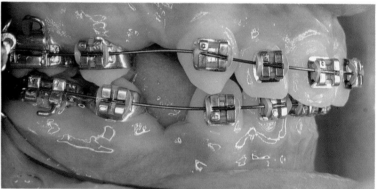

6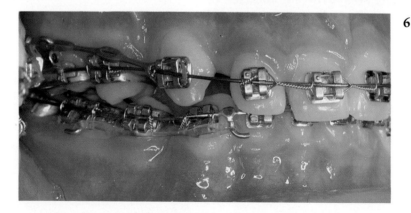

4-6 The treatment sequence above shows 'roller coaster' effect developing in an early treatment with the preadjusted appliance. The unwanted deepening of overbite was due to excess force, following attempts to transfer standard edgewise treatment mechanics and force levels to the new bracket system.

The Late 1970s

There were two possible ways to proceed. The route taken by Andrews (and later by Roth) was to maintain the same force levels and treatment mechanics, but introduce features into the bracket system to prevent undesirable changes. Hence, extra torque was introduced into incisor brackets and anti-tip and anti-rotation features were added to canine, premolar, and molar brackets. These were the 'extraction' or 'translation' series of brackets, some of which were later grouped together to produce the definitive Roth appliance.

An alternative route existed. This was taken by the authors, and it involved abandoning the traditional concepts of treatment mechanics. It required re-thinking the total force delivery system, with the new generation of brackets in mind. This required time, in contrast to the bracket modification alternative, which could be carried out very quickly. Such a system of force levels could only be developed on a basis of clinical trial and error, over a number of years, in the treatment of many hundreds of cases. This book presents a detailed overview of the authors' treatment philosophy, as it stands in 1992 following 12 years of development. It is currently employed by many colleagues who have adopted the treatment method.

The technique is offered as a treatment modality for the busy orthodontist, who is engaged in the day-to-day practice of clinical orthodontics. In the environment of private clinical practice, consistent high quality results are essential, with an efficient delivery system. Although this text is largely theoretical, it is supplemented with detailed step-by-step case reports, to demonstrate the mechanics in action, and emphasize the ease of treatment, the efficiency, and the consistent high quality of finished cases. A large number of color photographs have been included to complement and clarify the text, although space limitations allow inclusion only of a small number of case reports.

Orthodontists tend to have an independent outlook, and often wish to experiment or vary recommended techniques, seeking further improvement. It is the recommendation of the authors that any colleague who adopts this approach should avoid this temptation, at least for three years. Over the past 12 years they have clinically evaluated almost every conceivable variation, and this text represents the best of the alternatives.

Hopefully, those new to the technique will accept the whole philosophy in the first instance, including all the detail recommendations, before seeking to introduce their own variations for attempted improvement. The details are important, and careful adherence to the prescribed treatment protocol is recommended if one is to obtain a full measure of benefit from this treatment method.

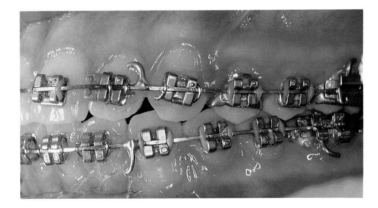

7

7 Andrews developed the Straight-Wire® Appliance with torque, tip and in/out built into each bracket. It became widely available in the 1970s, and was based on scientific measurements taken from 120 non-orthodontic normal cases.

2. TREATMENT MECHANICS:
A NEW APPROACH

Patience from the Orthodontist

Correct preadjusted appliance technique involves a gentle, progressive movement of teeth from a wrong position, to an ideal position. This should take place in a 'vectored' fashion, with each tooth and its root being translated into the correct position.

Undesirable tooth movements, such as excess crown tipping, will prevent achievement of the above, and it is therefore most important for the orthodontist to keep forces light, and to avoid trying to accelerate tooth movements.

During *leveling and aligning*, it is important to resist the temptation to 'race' through the archwires, and the cases show better progress if wires are not changed too frequently.

In *space closure* the elastic module on the tieback should not be stretched beyond twice its normal size. Usually, it is not helpful to increase force by the use of two modules, or other mechanisms, except sometimes at the end of space closure.

During *finishing* there is a tendency to cease treatment too early. Often the occlusion will continue to improve over a three-month period, by patiently re-tying the archwires carefully at each visit.

The .022 Slot versus .018 Slot

The appliance was originally designed for the .022 system and it seems to work best in this form. Many orthodontists have started with .018 and later switched into .022, finding the larger slot size to be better (8). The main advantages of the .022 system seem to be:

- Reduced treatment forces, especially during the opening stages. The larger slot allows more freedom for starting wires, and helps to keep force levels light.
- Working rectangular wires can be of .019/.025 and these seem to perform well during sliding mechanics and give good overbite control. With the .018 slot the main working wire is normally .017/.025. This wire is more flexible and hence shows greater deflection and binding during space closure with sliding mechanics (9).

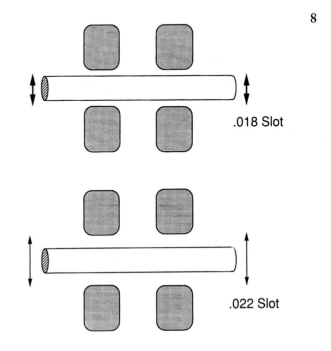

8

.018 Slot

.022 Slot

8 Line drawing to show starting .015 wire in .018 slot and .022 slot.

9

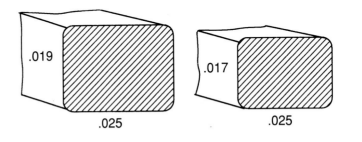

.019

.025

.017

.025

9 The .019/.025 rectangular working wire is more rigid than .017/.025 and provides better control during space closure.

Extraction Series Brackets

Andrews suggested a wide range of brackets as a further development of the basic Straight-Wire® Appliance, which he called 'Extraction' or 'Translation' brackets. These contained variations in tip, torque and rotation, designed to meet the needs of individual cases. In particular they were recommended to counteract tip and rotation changes during tooth movement when treating extraction cases.

While 'extraction series' brackets have theoretical advantages, it has been found that gentle forces, combined with the brackets recommended in Chapter 3, routinely achieve proper treatment goals. There are three main disadvantages to using extraction series brackets:

- Undesirable force vectors, (especially the tip on canines) are increased in the early stages of treatment.
- When light forces are used, the overcorrection built into extraction series brackets is not necessary.
- There is a need for substantially increased band and bracket inventory, or else a need to weld brackets at the chairside, with inherent possibilities of inaccuracy.

Power Arms

Power arms offer a mechanical advantage during canine retraction, because of the force application point being closer to the center of resistance of the tooth.

In practice they are not used as much as might be expected, and an orthodontist switching over to the Straight-Wire® Appliance may prefer to avoid using them for the first year or two. If power arms are to be used, force should not be applied until full bracket engagement in .018 round wire has been achieved. The elastic retraction force should be light (maximum 100 Gm), and the bracket should be tied in with a wire ligature.

The recommended mechanics require only a minimal retraction of canines, which are not retracted from the lateral incisors, but are moved only enough to allow good alignment of the six anterior teeth. These are then moved as a group 'en masse', with sliding mechanics and group tooth movement (**11**). This minimal canine retraction can usually be achieved using lacebacks, and hence the authors no longer have a need for power arms.

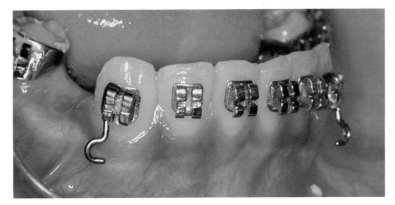

10 Power arms.

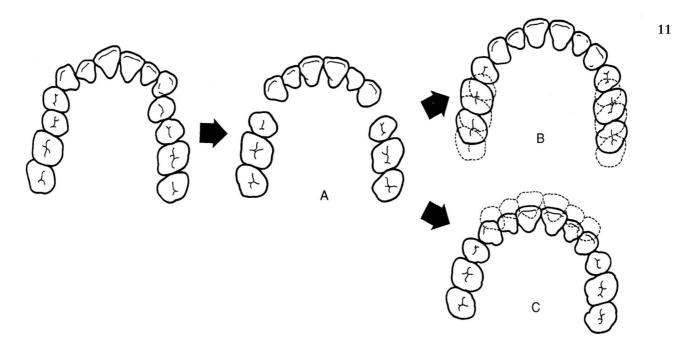

11 Canines are retracted only enough to allow alignment of the anterior teeth. This is followed by group movement and sliding mechanics.

Opening Archwires

12

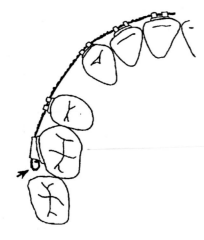

12 'Bendbacks' behind the most distally banded upper molars will establish control of upper incisors during early leveling and aligning with multistrand wires.

Recommended beginning archwires are .015 or .0175 multistrand. The forces at the *start* of treatment should be very light, and designed to minimize the demand on anchorage. It has been found that initially placing steel wires of .014 or .016 dimension gives forces which are too high.

Nickel titanium wires can be used, but they are expensive and there is a tendency to overextend them, away from the primary archform, because of their flexibility. This can produce unwanted changes in archform. It is recommended that opening archwires be contoured to an appropriate archform before placement. In many instances it is helpful to bend the ends of the opening wire into small circles immediately distal to the molar tube (especially the upper arch) to limit the arch length during leveling and aligning procedures. These 'bendbacks' are fully described in Chapter 7.

13

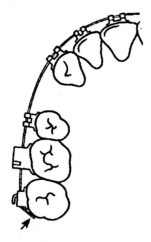

13 'Bendbacks' during later leveling and aligning with round wires are in the form of simple bends, after softening the wire, rather than the circles used with multistrand wires.

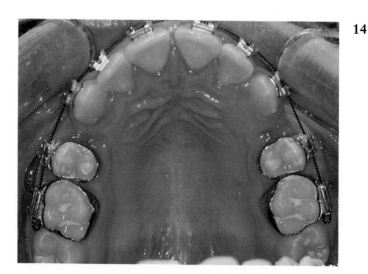

14

14 'Bendbacks' early in treatment.

Canine Lacebacks

These are constructed using .009 or .010 ligature wire and have proven extremely effective in controlling the canines during leveling and aligning.

The 11° of tip in a standard upper canine bracket will tend to throw the canine crown forward when an archwire is placed. This tendency is increased if an extraction series bracket is used, or if a heavy opening archwire is placed instead of .015 or .0175 multistrand.

Lacebacks are helpful when it is undesirable for canine crowns to tip mesially during leveling and aligning. In particular, this would apply to maxillary canines in Class II division 1 cases, and mandibular canines in Class III cases. It would apply to all canines in bimaxillary proclination cases.

They are placed prior to insertion of the initial archwire, and are often continued through the first few months of treatment. They should be passive, and not over-tightened. At routine monthly adjustment visits it is usually necessary to tighten each laceback, to take up 1 mm or so of slack, due to tooth movement. In maximum anchorage cases upper first molars may be supported with a palatal bar or with a headgear, to help anchorage control.

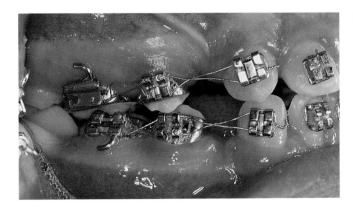

15 This bimaxillary proclination case carries lacebacks to canines to prevent mesial movement of crowns during leveling and aligning in response to opening wires. At routine monthly adjustment visits lacebacks are often 1 mm slack, and require gentle re-tightening to maintain control.

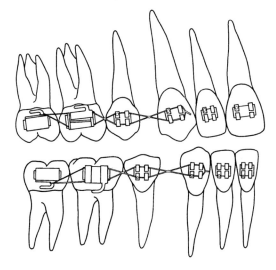

16 Lacebacks are placed prior to insertion of the initial archwire, and are often continued through the first few months of treatment. They should be passive, and not over-tightened.

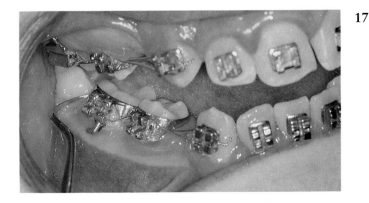

17 As a technique point, it may be found that the laceback tends to obscure the distal lumen of the molar tube, when carried to first molar bracket instead of second molar hook. This may be adjusted using a ligature director or an explorer.

Bracket and Band Positioning

18

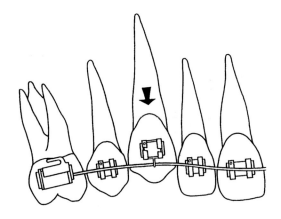

18 This canine has erupted sufficiently to be bracketed. At this appointment it will be necessary to drop to a flexible archwire, and therefore any incorrectly placed bands or brackets should be repositioned at this same visit.

The Straight-Wire® Appliance is a refined, precise system, and this precision needs to be reflected in appliance placement. Plenty of time should be allocated for setting up the case as accurately as possible. Care at this stage will be reflected later, in the quality of the result and in the efficiency of treatment. If a bracket or band is identified during treatment as being incorrectly placed, it should be repositioned. This is to be preferred to placing archwire bends. There are three convenient times for this:

- Before proceeding beyond the .014 round wire stage of leveling and aligning. The .014 round wire can be effectively used to 'step' teeth into a corrected position. The bracket can then be repositioned at the following visit.
- When picking up newly erupted teeth, such as canines or second molars. At this stage it is necessary to drop to a flexible wire, and it is convenient to change any incorrect brackets.
- If a patient arrives with a loose band or bracket at a normal adjustment visit and the tooth has shifted in position.

19

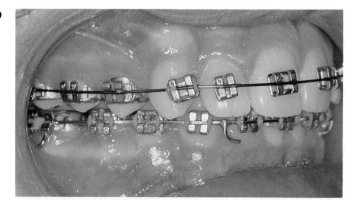

19 This patient arrived with a loose bracket, and the tooth had moved out of alignment. Any wrongly placed brackets should be repositioned at this visit also.

Banding and Bonding

It is generally recommended that molars and premolars be banded, with canines and incisors being bonded, in routine cases (20). Separation is essential in ensuring accurate band placement. It is possible to bond brackets onto premolars, but bands are generally stronger and more accurate. In adult cases, where access is good and the teeth have mature clinical crowns, bonding of premolars may be better, especially in non-extraction cases (21). It may be helpful to band rotated canines, and use lingual cleats to assist rotation control. It is useful to keep a small stock of incisor bands, upper and lower. These are sometimes needed for heavily restored or crowned teeth (22). Also, if a lower incisor bonded bracket is shed, it may be expedient to place a band, thereby avoiding the need to drop down an archwire size.

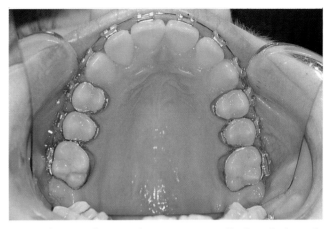

20 Molars and premolars are normally banded, and incisors and canines bonded, in routine treatment of youngsters.

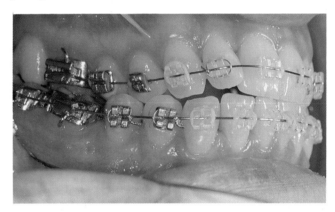

21 Adult cases often involve bonding of premolar brackets, especially in non-extraction treatments.

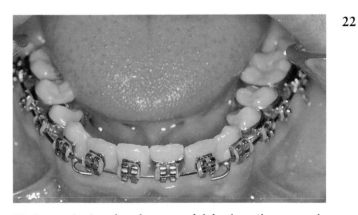

22 Lower incisor bands are useful for heavily restored teeth, or sometimes following shedding of a bonded bracket.

Stainless Steel Round Wires

23

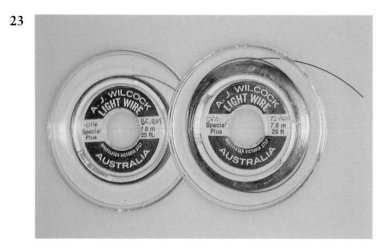

23 Special Plus round wires by A.J. Wilcock have proved effective in .014,.016,.018 and .020 wire sizes.

The round wires normally used are .014, .016, .018, and .020. They are used in the leveling and aligning phase, between multistrand wires and .019/.025 rectangular. Australian wires by A.J. Wilcock are particularly effective in cases with overbite problems, but any high quality stainless steel wire can prove to be satisfactory.

It is helpful to flame the distal 3 mm ends of steel archwires before placement, to allow for 'bendbacks'. These ensure patient comfort and limit arch length in leveling and aligning. They are used when it is desirable to maintain or decrease arch length. They are not used when increasing arch length, such as when expanding for non-extraction treatment. Softening the ends of round wires also allows easy removal at monthly adjustment visits.

One Size of Rectangular Wire

The preferred size of rectangular wire is .019/.025, to be used as the only size of rectangular wire in normal treatment. Larger, full thickness wires have been evaluated and they provide greater control, but are less effective for sliding mechanics, although .0215/.028 rectangular steel or nickel titanium wires may occasionally be considered in the final stages of treatment, to obtain maximal bracket expression.

It will normally be found that the change into .019/.025 rectangular wires can be made four to six weeks after placement of round .018 or .020 wires.

In cases which require a lot of leveling and aligning, it may be advisable to leave .020 wires in place longer, to allow for an easy, comfortable transition. There appears to be no advantage in an unduly rapid change from round to rectangular wires.

Theoretically there is approximately 10° of 'slop' or 'play' between .019/.025 wire and the .022 bracket slot (**24**), although in clinical use, the .019/.025 wire performs better than expected. This is probably due to the residual tip which remains uncorrected at the time of placement of rectangular wire. Thus, the situation as shown at **26** rather than **25** seems to more accurately represent the situation when rectangular wires are first placed.

The newly placed rectangular wire applies a commencing torque force at points X and Y. The forces are light, and comfortable for the patient.

24

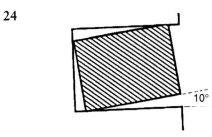

24 Approximately 10° of slop.

25

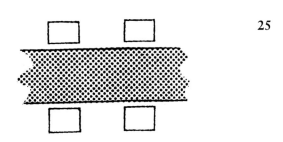

25 Theoretical arrangement at time of placement of rectangular wire.

26

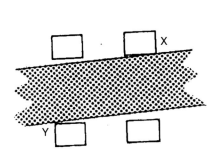

26 Actual arrangement at time of placement of rectangular wire, with tip which has not yet been corrected at X and Y.

27

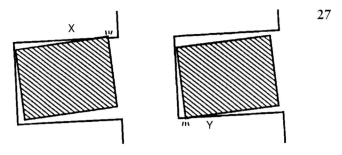

27 The newly placed rectangular wire applies a torque force at points X and Y. The forces are gentle, and comfortable for the patient.

The Use of Ligature Tying Pliers

It is logical for the orthodontist to seek to obtain as much performance as possible from a precise, accurate bracket system.

Elastomeric modules are normally used for attachment of the archwire during the early stages of treatment, to reduce force levels and encourage free movement of teeth. The modules may be 'worked' a little on the cane before placement, to ease handling. The option of colored modules is popular with some younger patients and this may be used to encourage good oral hygiene with the words 'Yes, you may have colored elastics when you show a good standard of brushing'. Rectangular wires are normally placed using elastic modules for the first one or two months. After that, ligature-tying pliers may be used with .010 ligature wires, to ensure more positive archwire engagement into the bracket slot. Also, during the closing stages of treatment, it often enhances the result if the appliance is kept in place for an extra two or three months, with brackets being re-tied every month.

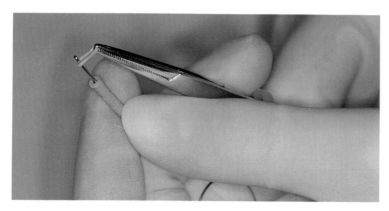

28 Modules may be worked on the cane before placement, to ease handling.

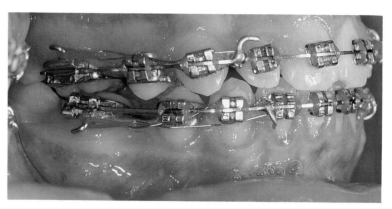

29 Colored modules are popular with some younger patients and may be offered as an incentive towards good tooth brushing.

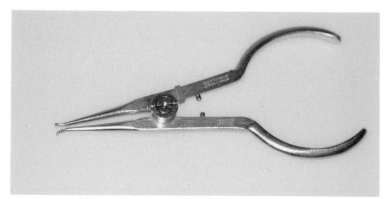

30 Coon Ligature-Tying Plier.

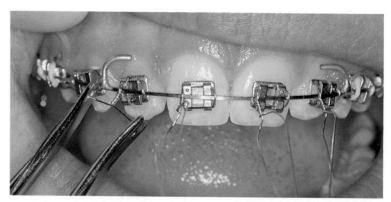

31 Tying in with wire ligatures, using Coon pliers, encourages full expression of the bracket system.

Standardized Archform

It is essential to use an appropriate archform. The archform used by the authors is slightly expanded in the bicuspid region to allow for proper functional movements and is close to the 'Roth' archform.

The archform shown in **32** has been in extensive clinical use for 12 years. It has proven appropriate for more than 80% of cases. Some adjustment may be needed in the remaining 20% of cases. Often this modification is merely a change in size, maintaining the same shape (**34, 34**).

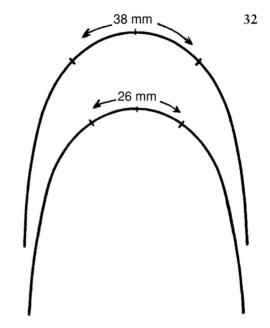

32 Standard archform, showing average positions for soldered hooks on rectangular wires. This form is used, unmodified, in more than 80% of cases.

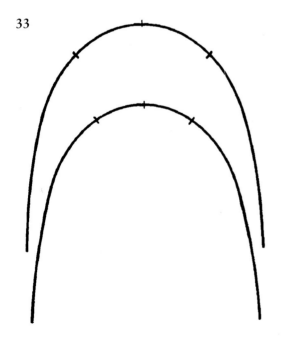

33 Standard archform plus 5%.

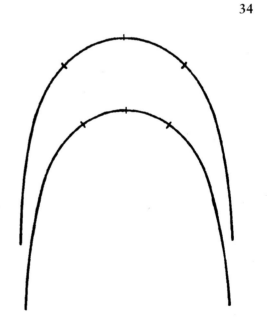

34 Standard archform minus 5%.

Rotation Control

It is fundamental that tooth rotation should be controlled without archwire bends if possible. The brackets are 'twin' type and this allows quite good control from the buccal side. Additionally, lingual cleats or wedges may be used.

Lingual cleats are useful in controlling rotation of molars, premolars and canines, whereas Steiner metal wedges are effective on all teeth, except where the bracket has a large element of tip built into it. With canines and upper lateral incisors, for example, metal wedges are not effective. It is necessary to reduce one wing of the Steiner wedge for optimal effectiveness with lower incisors.

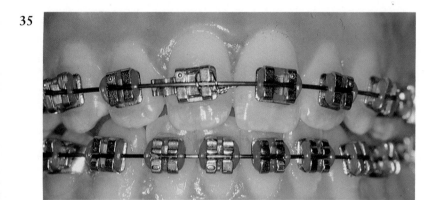

35 Steiner metal wedges are effective on all teeth, except where the bracket has a large element of tip built into it. The wedge is placed before or after insertion of the archwire, and in this case it was placed before. These metal wedges do not deteriorate in the same way as rubber wedges and seldom need to be replaced.

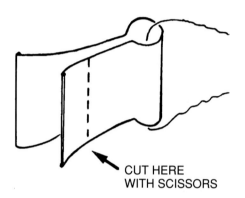

CUT HERE
WITH SCISSORS

36 It is helpful to reduce one wing of the Steiner wedge, as shown, for use with lower incisors.

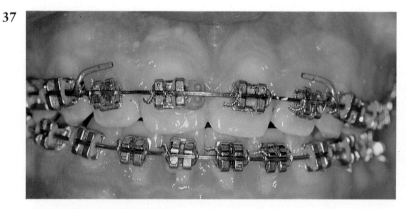

37 Rubber rotation wedges work very well with the Straight-Wire® Appliance, irrespective of how much tip is built-in. They are added to one wing of the bracket prior to archwire placement.

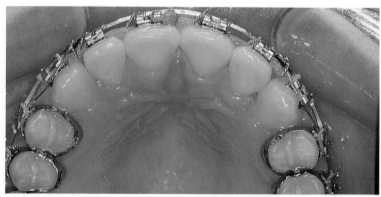

38 It is important, when a rubber rotation wedge is placed on one wing of the bracket, to make sure that the other wing is firmly tied with a wire ligature.

Sliding Mechanics

One of the main advantages of the Straight-Wire® Appliance is that it achieves true level slot line-up. This, in turn, allows sliding mechanics and group movement of teeth (39). Space closure is achieved by using a 'tieback' to deliver a force between the molar bracket (first or second molar) and the soldered archwire hook.

A normal elastic module is stretched to twice its resting size,

and there are two common arrangements for this (40, 41).

It is often asked 'Why not simply stretch a chain of modules from hook to hook?' This, and many other methods have been tried. A chain does not give a precise force, it is more difficult to clean, and it sometimes falls off. It is recommended that one of the tieback methods displayed here should be used (see also 43 and 44 on the following page).

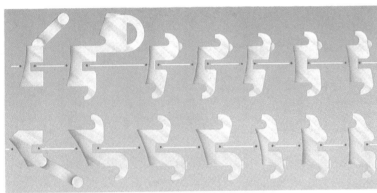

39 Level slot line-up of all teeth allows sliding mechanics and group movement of teeth.

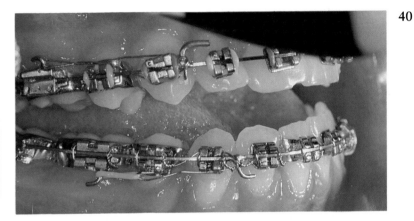

40 An example of a tieback for lower space closure, with the module on the molar hook. A colored module has been used for clarity, but normally gray modules are used.

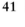
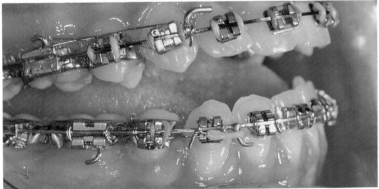

41 An example of a tieback for lower space closure, with the module on the archwire hook. Colored modules have been used for clarity, but normally gray modules are used. The principle and the force level is the same as in 40.

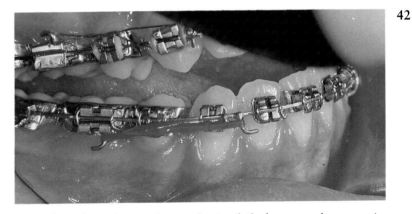

42 Asking the patient to change elastics daily for space closure, as in Stage II Begg treatment, relies on good co-operation which is not always forthcoming.

43

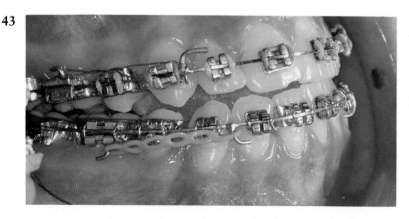

44

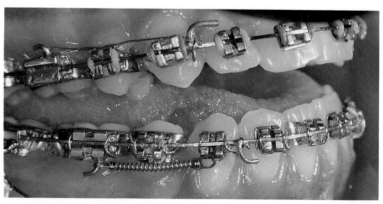

43 Stretching a chain of modules between the hooks gives an inconsistent force. The chain is difficult to clean and it somtimes falls off.

44 Recent research has shown encouraging results from the use of nickel titanium coil springs, which seem to show more consistent and slightly more rapid tooth translation. This method is fully described in Chapter 10.

Archwire Bends

45

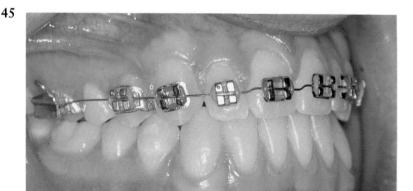

45 During the final weeks of treatment it is sometimes helpful to place .014 steel wires to achieve good inter-cuspation. Partial band and bracket removal was carried out two weeks prior to this photograph.

In the later stages of each treatment it is necessary to place bends in the archwires, and these are discussed in Chapter 11. It is not correct to assume that the Straight-Wire® Appliance will achieve full correction without any archwire bends. The situation has been compared to a journey of five miles. The appliance will take care of the first four and a half miles, but then it is necessary to walk the remaining half mile.

It is normally correct to place initial rectangular wires in a flat, unmodified form. Archwire bends are then introduced, as needed, when wires have been in place for one to three months to ensure passivity.

Archwire bends should not normally be introduced to compensate for a wrongly placed bracket. It is better to replace the band or bonded bracket. During the final weeks of treatment it is sometimes helpful to place .014 steel wires to achieve good inter-cuspation. These are comfortable for the patient and easily adjusted by the orthodontist.

CASE REPORT SB

A Class I four bicuspid extraction case

This 15 year old girl presented with a Class I skeletal and dental pattern. She showed an average lower facial height, with moderate protrusion of upper and lower incisors, which resulted in her lips being apart at rest.

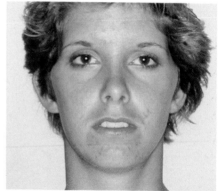

46

There was moderate crowding in the upper and lower anterior segments, and as a result, it was decided to extract four first premolars.

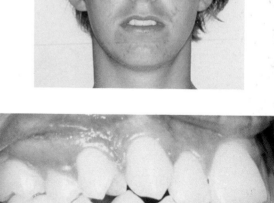

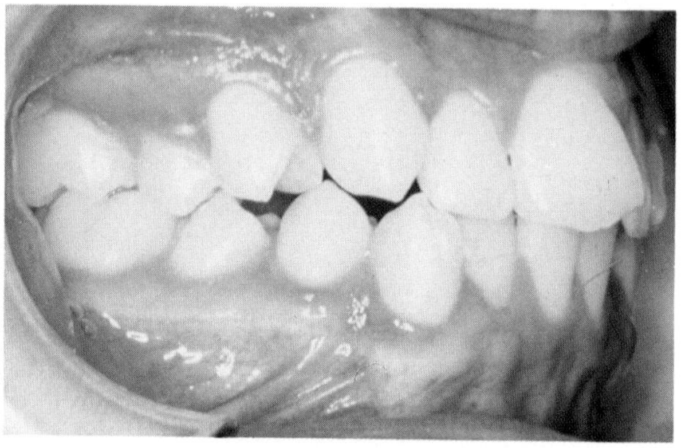

49

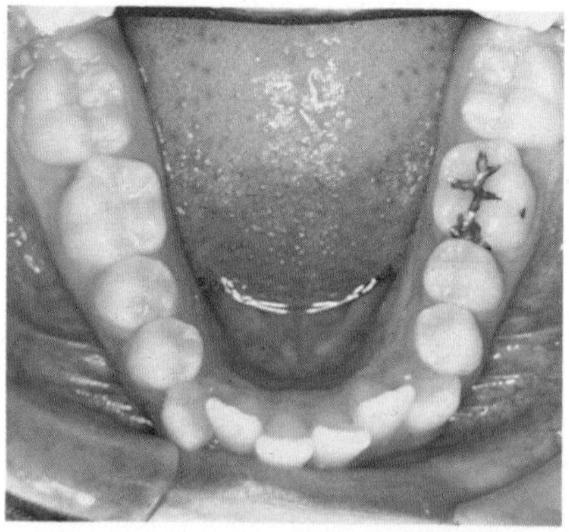

52

The case was managed as a minimal anchorage treatment, with no use of headgear, lingual arches, or palatal bars.

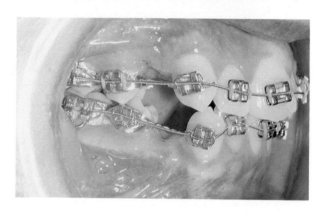

55

47

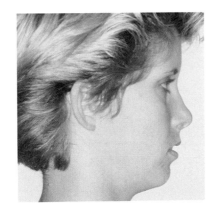

48

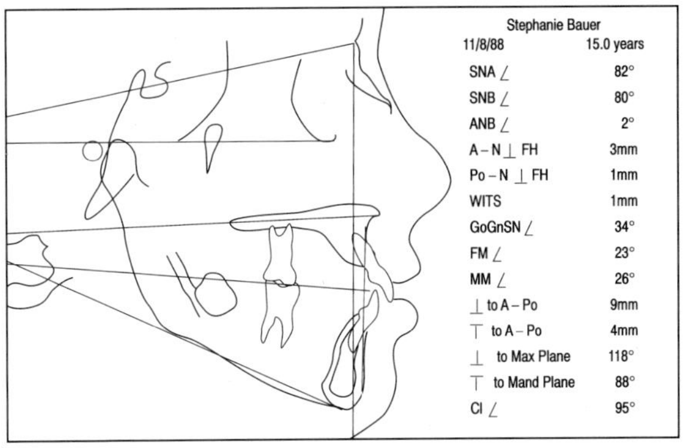

	Stephanie Bauer	
	11/8/88	15.0 years
SNA ∠		82°
SNB ∠		80°
ANB ∠		2°
A – N ⊥ FH		3mm
Po – N ⊥ FH		1mm
WITS		1mm
GoGnSN ∠		34°
FM ∠		23°
MM ∠		26°
⊥ to A – Po		9mm
⊤ to A – Po		4mm
⊥ to Max Plane		118°
⊤ to Mand Plane		88°
CI ∠		95°

50

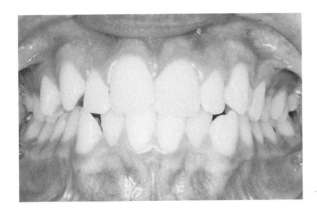

51

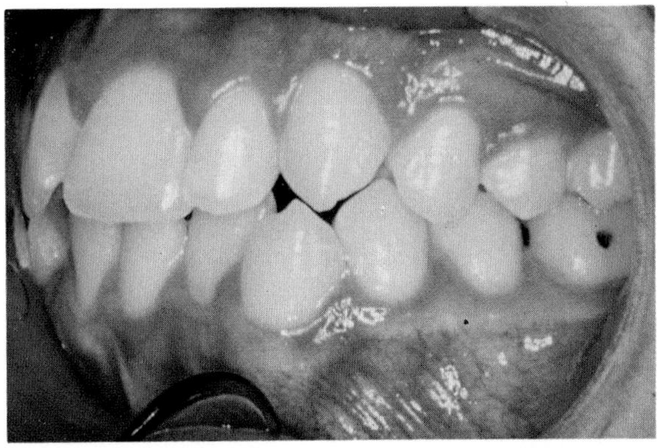

53

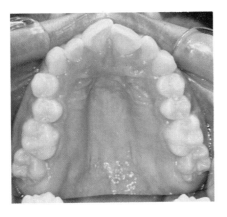

54

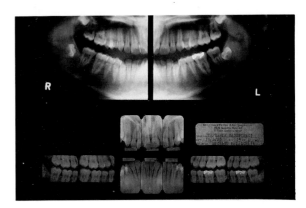

56

INITIAL LEVELING STAGE

1 **Brackets on all possible teeth**
2 **Standard appliance (.022)**
3 **Lacebacks to cuspids**
  a **Anchorage support**
4 **Initial wire 15 TF**
  a **Bendbacks for incisors**
  b **Patience — hold crowns, let roots move**
5 **Wire sequence**
  a **15 TF 17 TF**
  b **.014 .016 .018 .020 round**

57

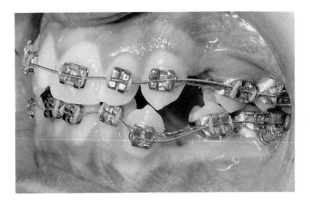

Bendbacks were used in both arches, and canines were controlled with lacebacks.

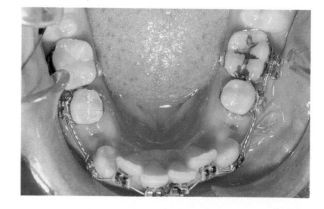

58

After two months of treatment, with .014 round wires in place.

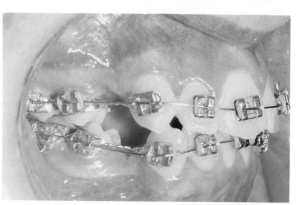

61

Lacebacks and bendbacks continue to control canines and incisors.

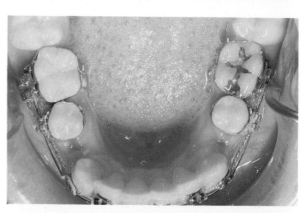

64

After three months of treatment.

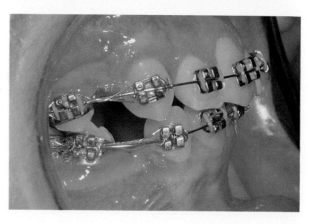

66

59

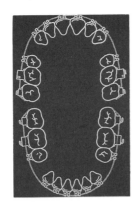

60

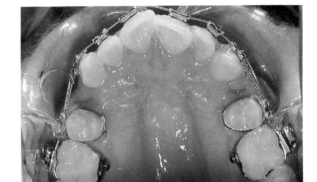

62

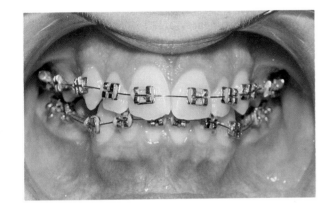

63

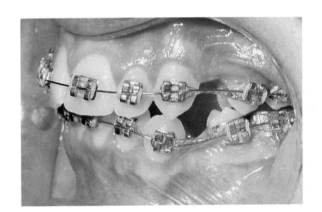

65

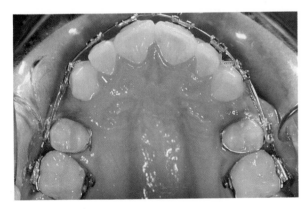

67

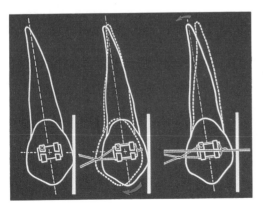

68

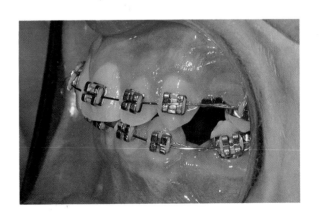

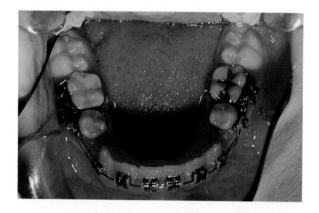

An upper .019/.025 rectangular wire is in place, with passive tiebacks. In the lower arch a round wire is continuing leveling and aligning, without lacebacks, to avoid canine retraction away from the lateral incisors.

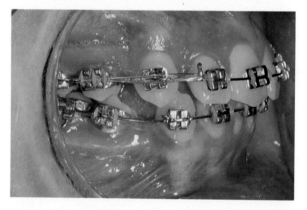

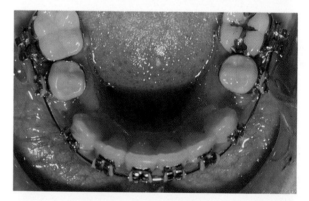

Start of upper and lower space closure with active tiebacks to elastic modules, using the hooks on the rectangular wires.

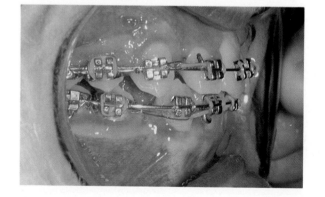

70
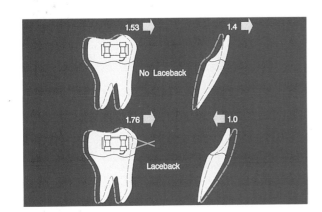

71
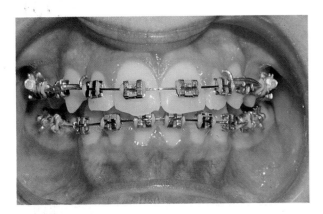

73
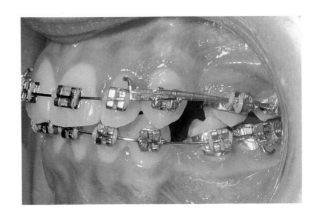

74
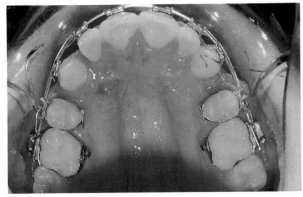

76
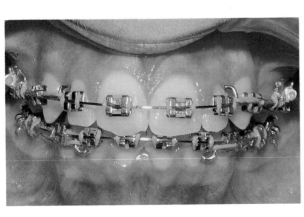

78
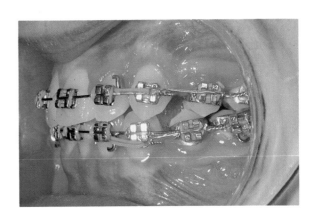

79

Fourteen months into treatment, and continuing space closure. Adjustment visits are short at this stage.

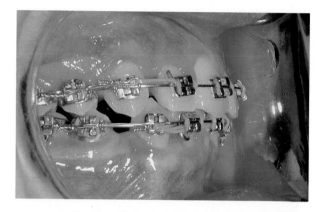

80

One elastic module is normally enough, but sometimes two may be used.

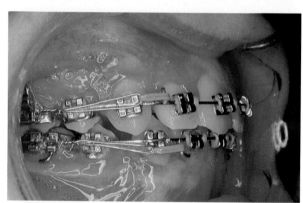

83

Occlusal views show the effect of sliding mechanics, giving efficient space closure. Second molars will be banded later, after space closure.

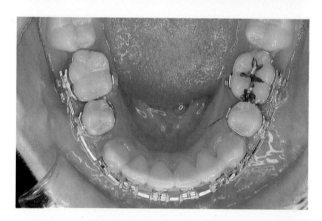

86

At completion of space closure, passive tiebacks are used to hold the spaces closed. Modules can be placed over the tiebacks, to stabilize them, and help oral hygiene.

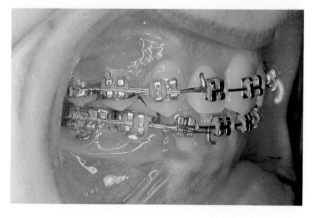

88

81
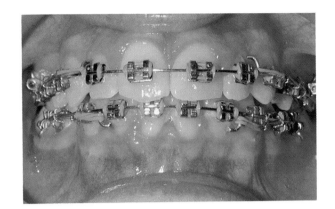

82
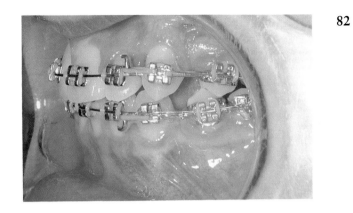

84
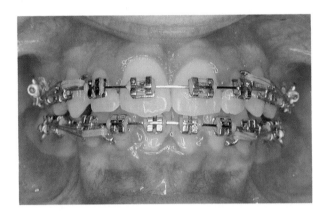

85
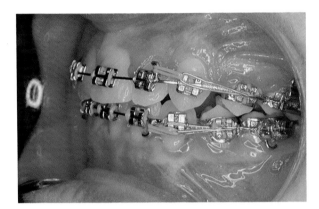

87
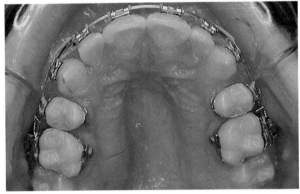

89
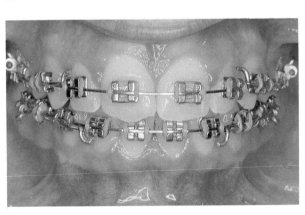

90
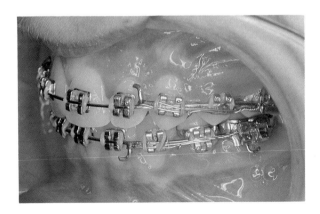

Re-leveling using .014 round wires after banding the upper and lower second molars. Careful bendbacks are needed to prevent spaces re-opening, or else lacebacks may be used.

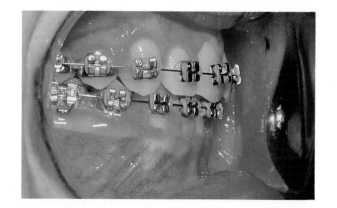

91

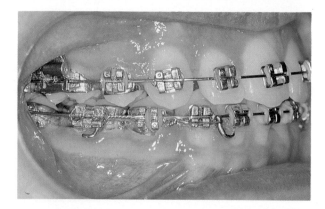

94

Close to the end of treatment. Upper and lower .019/.025 rectangular wires, with a passive lower tieback. The active upper tieback is being used to finally close extraction space.

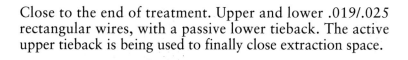
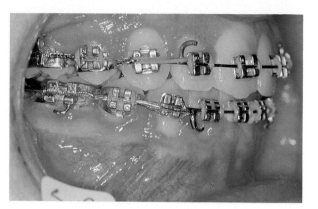

97

92

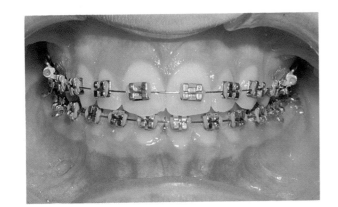

93

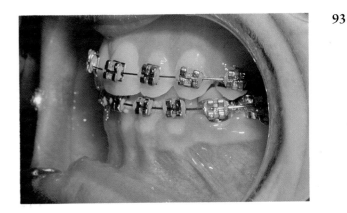

95

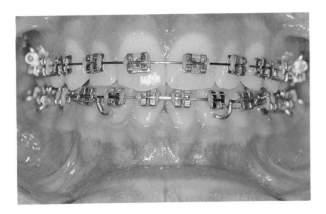

96

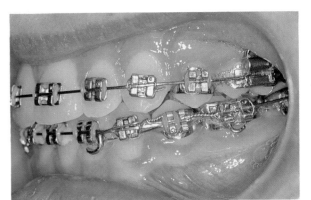

98

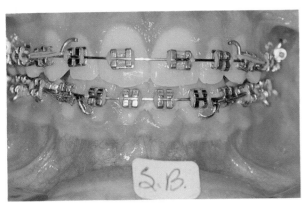

99

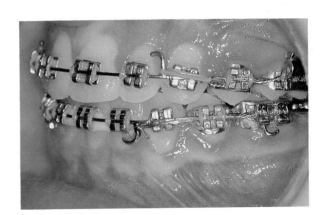

Active treatment time was 19 months.

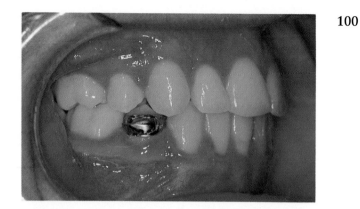

100

A nocturnal upper Hawley retainer was worn, and a lower fixed retainer. The gray color of the lower incisor is a photographic artefact, and the tooth was quite healthy.

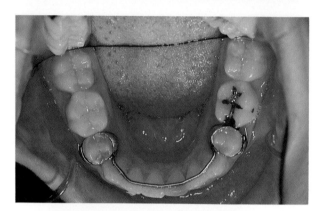

103

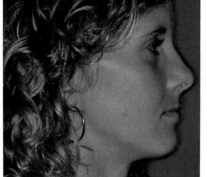

106

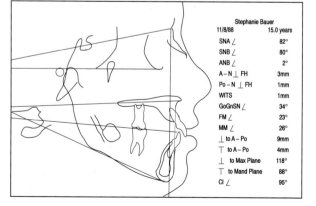

109

101

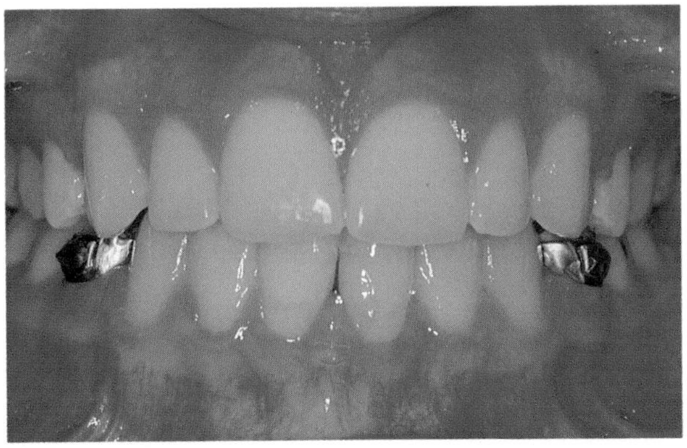

102

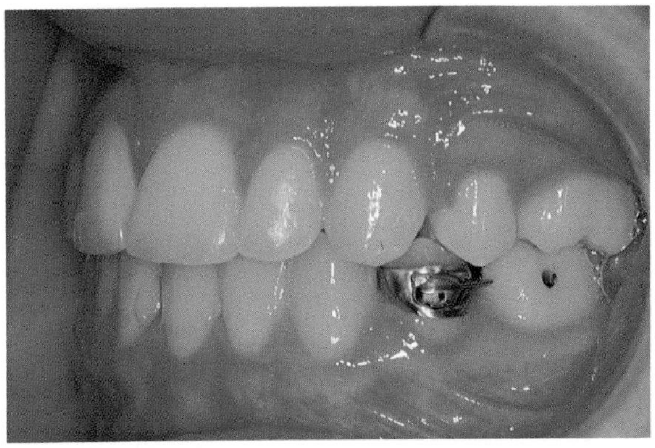

104

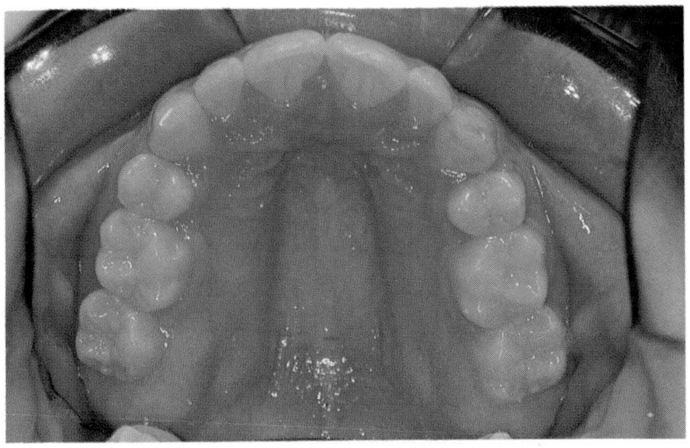

105

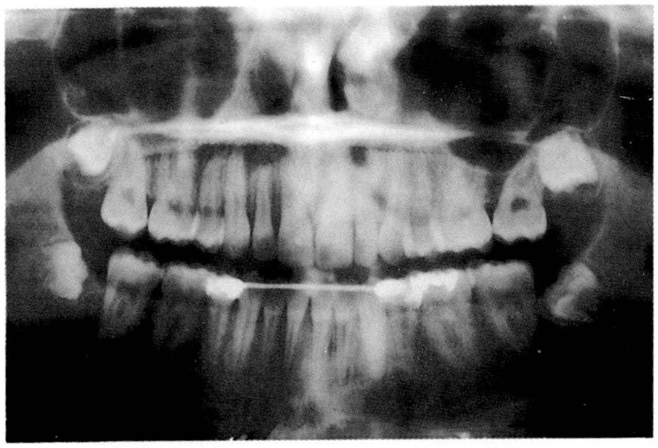

107

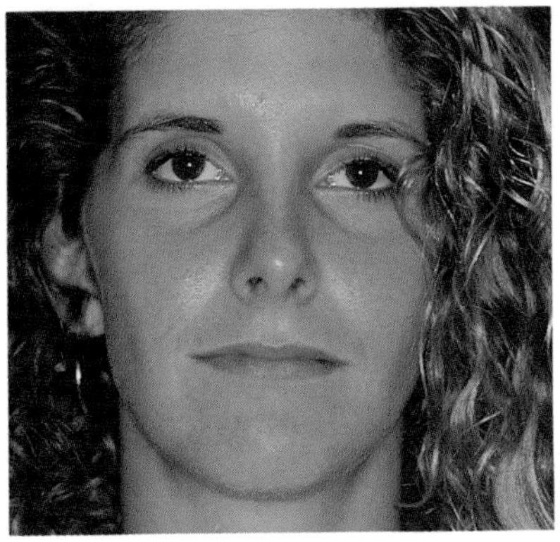

108

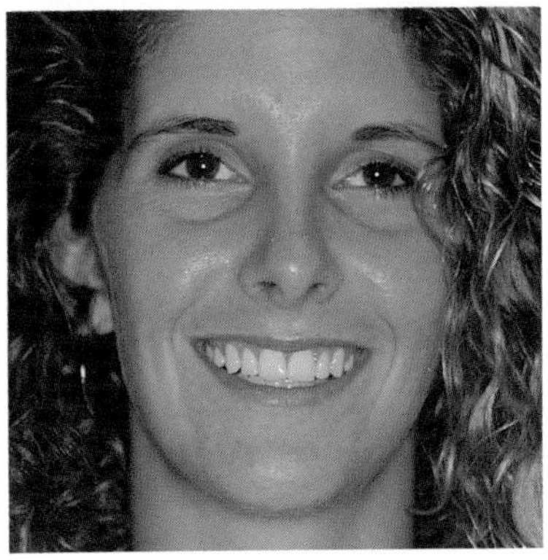

110

111

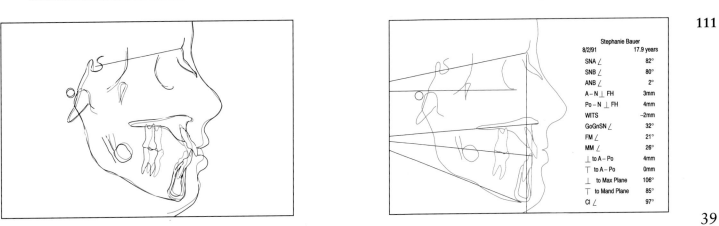

Stephanie Bauer	
8/2/91	17.9 years
SNA ∠	82°
SNB ∠	80°
ANB ∠	2°
A – N ⊥ FH	3mm
Po – N ⊥ FH	4mm
WITS	–2mm
GoGnSN ∠	32°
FM ∠	21°
MM ∠	26°
⊥ to A – Po	4mm
⊤ to A – Po	0mm
⊥ to Max Plane	106°
⊤ to Mand Plane	85°
CI ∠	97°

3. APPLIANCE SELECTION: RECOMMENDED SPECIFICATIONS

Background

Since the mid-1970s the authors have worked to develop and refine treatment mechanics appropriate to the new generation of preadjusted edgewise appliances. In 1989, a preliminary report on this method of treatment mechanics was published in the *Journal of Clinical Orthodontics*.[1]

While developing an effective mechanical approach and establishing ideal force levels, the authors have used primarily the standard Straight-Wire® Appliance,[2] as well as a number of bracket and tube variations of that appliance. The use of this wide range of brackets and tubes in numerous clinical situations has allowed the development of an appliance system that has worked most effectively with the recommended mechanics. Before going into a detailed description of this appliance system, it is helpful to make a few general comments concerning the development of the appliance.

The original standard 'straight wire' appliance was a hybrid twin edgewise appliance with built in tip, torque and in-out measurements, derived from a set of 120 untreated but 'ideal' or 'normal' study models.[3] It also had secondary features added for ease of treatment and handling such as an identification system, extended gingival tie wings, convertible tubes, and contoured bracket bases. After the appliance was used for a period of time, three important facts became apparent:

- The 120 non-orthodontic normals generally showed broad, rounded dental bases, and the average measurements were appropriate for cases with underlying bone structure of that type. In contrast, many orthodontic cases presented with narrowed maxillary and mandibular bone.
- While most patients' teeth approach the shape of those on the untreated study models, there was enough variation with some individuals to either require wire bending during the finishing stages of treatment or the development of additional brackets with variations in the amount of tip, torque and in-out compensation.
- The standard appliance measurements were based on static tooth positions and in all cases did not adequately control the compensation required during the *movement* of teeth from one position to another. As a result of these factors, additional brackets were made available to either supplement or replace the standard straight-wire appliance.

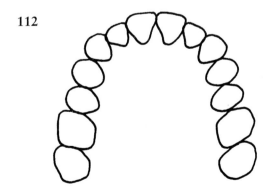

112 The non-orthodontic normal models typically were of individuals with broad, rounded dental bases.

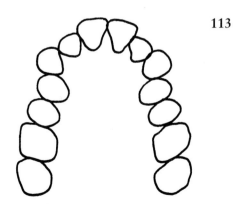

113 Many orthodontic cases present with narrowed maxillary and mandibular bone.

Bracket Development

The range of brackets has grown steadily over the years to meet the needs of a variety of orthodontists with different mechanical methods of treatment.

In addition to the demand for variations in bracket specifications (tip, torque and in-out), there developed a demand for different bracket shapes, designs and even materials. It was not long before a single wing bracket system was developed for users of that system.

The demand for a smaller and more comfortable bracket led to the production of the 'Attract'™ and 'Minitwin' brackets, while the additional demand for a more esthetic bracket led to the development of 'Starfire'™ brackets. Today the orthodontist has the opportunity to develop an appliance system within his practice to meet his own needs relative to his treatment mechanics, as well as to meet the specific priorities of his patients.

Appliance Selection Factors

With this wide variety of brackets has come the difficult task of selecting the most appropriate appliance system. The following factors need to be considered when making this important decision:

- The need for a practical and economical inventory size.
- The treatment mechanics and the force levels used during treatment.
- The willingness on the part of the orthodontist to place bends in the archwires during the finishing stages of treatment, as opposed to placing alternative brackets, to try to eliminate the need for those bends.

The authors have spent a great deal of time and effort in evaluating the most appropriate appliance system to use with their mechanics. This section describes, in detail, a system which will provide a basis for colleagues wishing to use the same mechanics, allowing them to make an easy choice from the bewildering range of available brackets. The authors accept that some recommended specifications could be varied or substituted without detracting from the efficiency of the mechanical approach. However, experience has shown that the details are important, and that certain key features must be considered as essential:

- Slot size .022/.028.
- Twin bracket system.
- All brackets to be crown related, with torque-in-base.
- First molar tubes to be convertible into brackets.
- Each first and second molar attachment to carry a hook.
- Headgear .045 tube to be gingival on upper first molars.

There is a built-in identification system for premolar, canine and incisor brackets, with dots on disto-gingival tie-wings in the upper, and dashes in the lower. All second premolar brackets have a cross on their mesio-gingival tie-wings. Attachments carry a built-in element of 'in-out', to reflect the different thickness of the teeth. Lacebacks are routinely used to retract canines just enough to allow alignment of the six anterior teeth, and therefore power arms are not used.

Recommended Specifications

Uppers

	7	6	5	4	3	2	1
Non-orthodontic normal values	Tip torque 5/–9	Tip torque 5/–9	Tip torque Same	Tip torque Same	Tip torque Same	Tip torque 9/3	Tip torque 5/7
Recommended Specifications	**0/–9**	**0/–9**	**2/–7**	**2/–7**	**11/–7**	**9/10**	**5/17**

rotation 10   rotation 10

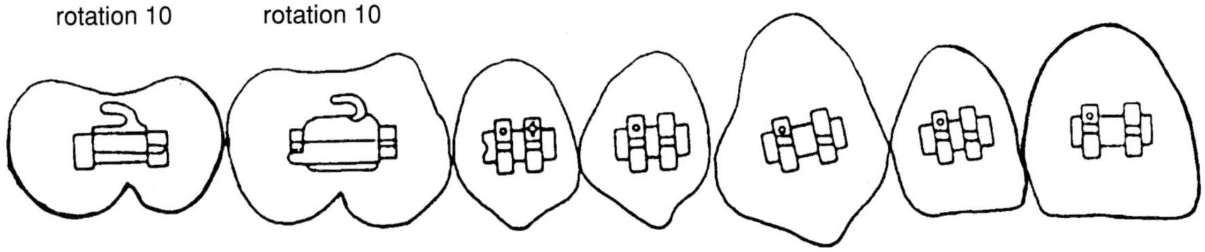

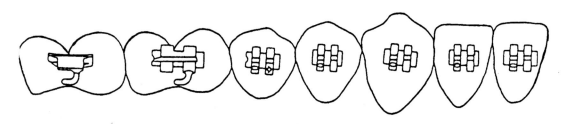

114

	7	6	5	4	3	2	1
Recommended Specifications	**2/–10**	**2/–26**	**2/–22**	**2/–17**	**5/–11**	**2/-6**	**2/–6**
Non-orthodontic normal values	2/–35 Tip torque	Same Tip torque	Same Tip torque	Same Tip torque	Same Tip torque	2/–1 Tip torque	2/–1 Tip torque

Lowers

Upper and Lower Incisors

Reason for changes from the non-orthodontic normal values

Upper incisors

	7	6	5	4	3	2	1
Non-orthodontic normal values						Tip torque 9/3	Tip torque 5/7
Recommended Specifications						**9/10**	**5/17**

115

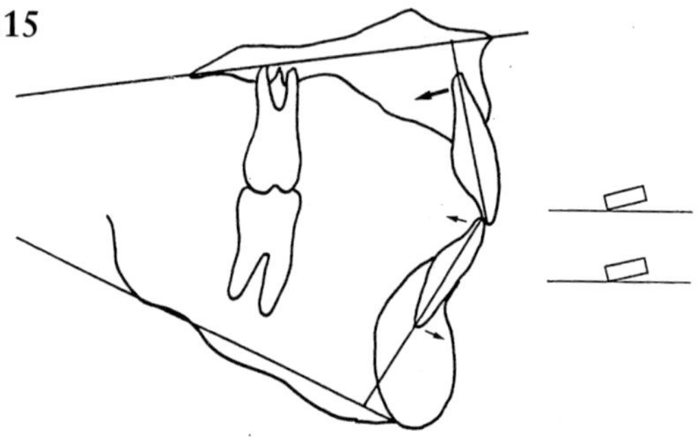

116

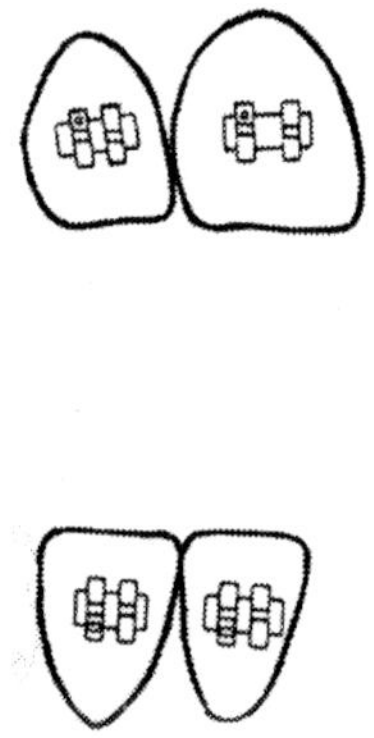

115–116 Wire bending of this type is needed less frequently if upper and lower incisor brackets of the recommended specification are used, rather than values from the non-orthodontic normals.

	7	6	5	4	3	2	1
Recommended Specifications						**2/–6**	**2/–6**
Non-orthodontic normal values						2/–1 Tip torque	2/–1 Tip torque

Lower incisors

Over the years the authors have found themselves 'adding torque' to rectangular wires in a high percentage of cases, seeking to achieve palatal root torque for the upper incisors and labial root torque for lower incisors, as shown in the figure above. Changing upper bracket torque by 10° for the central incisor and 7° for the lateral incisor, and lower bracket torque by 5° reduces the amount of wire bending required. Such brackets are especially helpful in the manage-ment of starting overjets in excess of 10 mm, Class II division 2 malocclusions, and routine Class II treatment which is being treated to an end-result with a residual Class II dental base discrepancy. The authors accept that there will often be a need to adjust incisor torque in rectangular wires, irrespective of the bracket specification, because at the start of treatment it is not possible to accurately predict the torque needs of a case some 18 months later.

Upper First and Second Molars

Reason for changes from the non-orthodontic normal values

Upper first and second molars

	7	6	5	4	3	2	1
Non-orthodontic normal values	Tip torque 5/–9	Tip torque 5/–9					
Recommended Specifications	**0/–9**	**0/–9**					

rotation 10   rotation 10

117

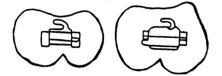

118 Upper molars are normally banded. If the 5/–9 brackets are used, it is necessary to place the bands at 5° to the buccal cusps, in order to get the bracket wings parallel with the buccal groove of the tooth. Bands do not fit in this position and it is difficult to routinely place them in this way.

119 The authors have found it preferable to use 0/–9 brackets and place the molar bands parallel with the buccal cusps of the molars because the bands fit much better in this position. This introduces the proper 5° of tip.

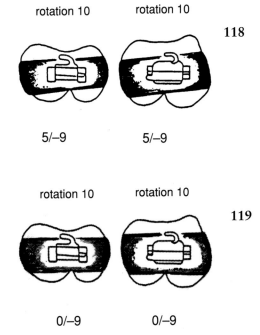

rotation 10   rotation 10   118

5/–9   5/–9

rotation 10   rotation 10   119

0/–9   0/–9

Lower Second Molar

Reason for changes from the non-orthodontic normal values

120
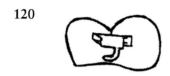

	7	6	5	4	3	2	1
Recommended Specifications	**2/–10**						
Non-orthodontic normal values	2/–35 Tip torque						

121
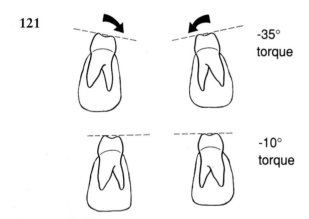

-35°
torque

-10°
torque

During treatment the authors have found a consistent tendency for lower second molars to roll lingually when using 2/–31 or even 2/–20 brackets. This molar rolling-in can come from three possible causes:

- Tube height inaccuracy between first and second molars.
- Archform effect, if it is unduly narrowed distal to the lower first molars.
- 'Plunger' effect of upper second molar cusps.

They have found the use of a 2/–10 specification helpful in controlling the lower second molar torque.

122
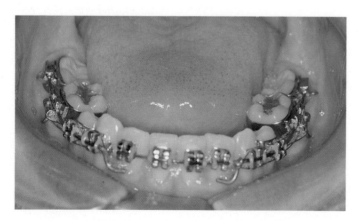

122 This tendency to rolling in of lower second molars can be controlled by using 2/–10 specification brackets.

4. APPLIANCE VARIATIONS

Introduction

A typical orthodontic caseload will involve the treatment of a high percentage of children, who will normally start correction before the age of fourteen. For these individuals there is a need to have the best possible tooth control, for a high quality result in a reasonably short treatment time, and the authors favor the use of metal twin appliances, as previously described in Chapter 3. There may be different priorities in some cases, and an alternative bracket prescription may be considered, due to one of the following:

- Treatment preference. The orthodontist wanting to change bracket prescription to help the planned treatment mechanics, and to minimize wire bending.
- Patient preference. A patient wanting more comfortable or more esthetic appliances.

There should be a balance between the patient's wishes, and the need for adequate control, because the choice of smaller or more esthetic brackets brings with it a reduction in tooth control. In a complicated case this may in turn lead to an increase in treatment time, or some kind of compromise in the end result, or both, compared with what could have been achieved with normal twin brackets. There is a need to fully discuss and explain this prior to starting treatment. In management of the most severe problems, such as those requiring orthognathic surgery, the orthodontist should firmly insist on maximal control, using twin metal brackets. More comfortable or more esthetic brackets may be considered with easier cases, especially if the treatment is non-extraction in type, without a need to control rotations or achieve big torque changes.

Treatment Preferences

Andrews[1] has favored a 'fully programmed' appliance régime, where an individualized twin bracket system is fitted for each patient, selecting from a relatively large range of possibilities. The intention of this approach is to fit a bracket prescription which will allow completion of treatment to full correction with an absolute minimum of wire bending.

The recommendation by Andrews represents the ultimate expression of 'treatment preference'. It requires careful treatment planning and individualized bracket selection before placing the appliance and starting tooth movements, in the anticipation that less wire bending will be needed to achieve those movements. Although it is logical, this idealistic approach has not seen widespread acceptance, for two reasons. Firstly, it has not proved possible to accurately predict growth, or correctly anticipate torque needs for individual cases some 18–24 months before starting treatment. Secondly, there are day-to-day practical difficulties in stocking a very wide range of brackets, and in welding them to bands, or bonding them to teeth. The authors, like Roth, have therefore settled for a bracket specification which is good for a high percentage of cases using their treatment mechanics, and they accept that some wire bending will be needed. They prefer to work with the brackets described in Chapter 3 on most routine treatments, but sometimes they will consider one of the following variations, depending on the nature of the starting malocclusion.

123

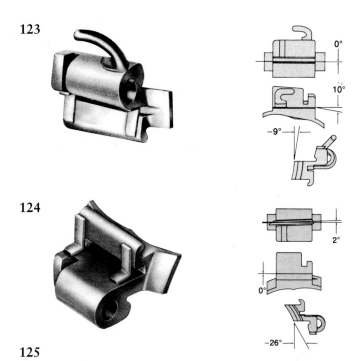

Malocclusion needing headgear

If it is intended to carry headgear to the upper first molars, an extra .045 tube for the inner bow is required. The headgear tube is gingival, to apply the force close to the center of resistance of the tooth (**123**).

124

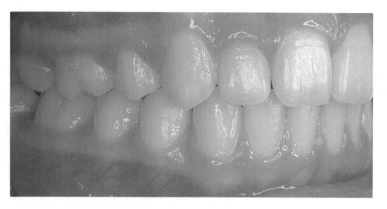

Lip bumper for distalizing lower molars

If it is intended to use a lip bumper for gaining lower arch space, there is a need for a special attachment for lower first molars. The tube in **124** carries an extra tube for the lip bumper.

125

Class II molar result

If it is intended to treat to a Class II molar result (for example, following loss of two upper premolars and no lower premolar extractions), then better occlusion can be obtained if upper first and second molars are allowed to rotate mesially. Occlusal adjustment may be required at the end of treatment to ensure good lateral excursions (**125, 126**).

125 Photo of Class II molar result.

126

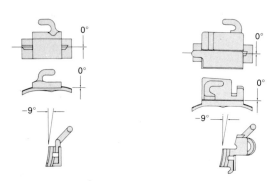

126 These tubes have zero distal rotation compared with 10° in a normal prescription. They are helpful when treating to a Class II molar result

Narrow maxillary or mandibular bone, needing different canine brackets

In contrast with the non-orthodontic normal models, which were taken from individuals with broad arches, the routine orthodontic patient often has narrow arches, with upper and lower canines blocked out buccally. Canine brackets with −7° upper torque and −11° lower torque are not helpful in correcting such problems. Often as the crowns of the canines are guided palatally, the roots can tend to stay labially placed. They are then in contact with the buccal cortical plate, and are difficult to retract. Canine brackets with zero torque encourage canine roots to lie more in cancellous bone, allowing easier retraction (see **131–135** on the following page).

127

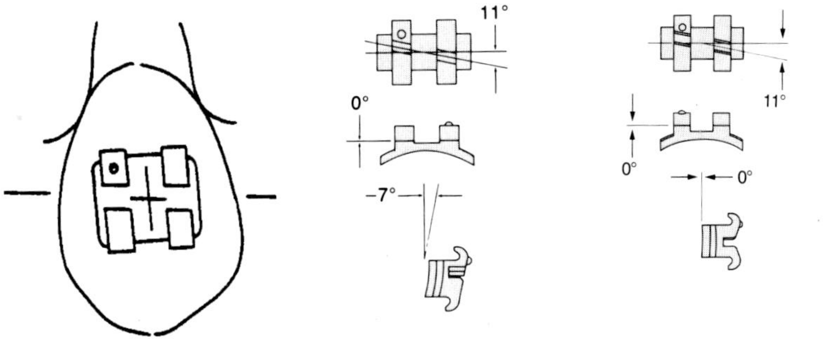

128

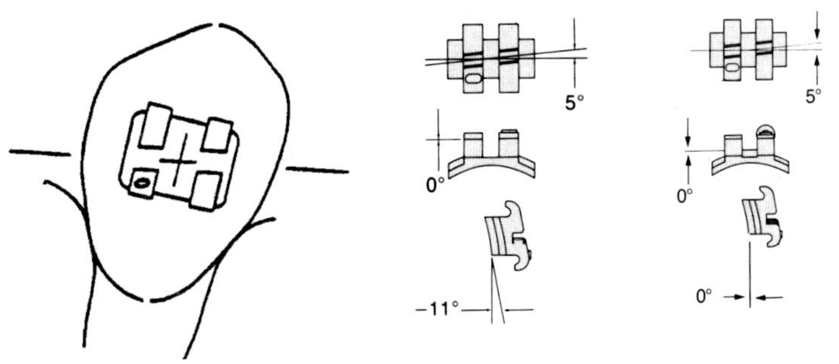

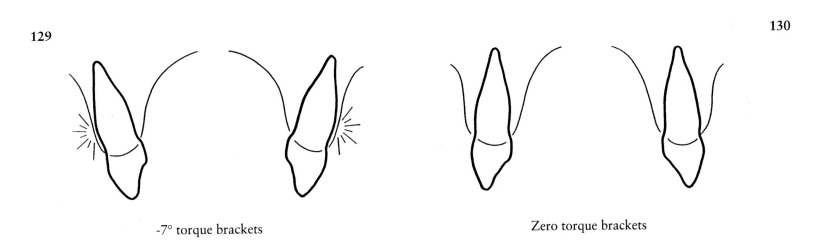

127 Upper canine brackets with a zero torque specification can be helpful in the management of cases with narrow maxillary bone. The canine roots tend to lie in away from the cortical plate, in cancellous bone, and can be moved much more easily.

128 Lower canine brackets with a zero torque specification can be helpful in the management of cases with narrow mandibular bone.

129

130

-7° torque brackets

Zero torque brackets

129–130 Upper canine brackets with zero torque can help to keep the canine roots away from the cortical plate, in cancellous bone, and they can be moved much more easily.

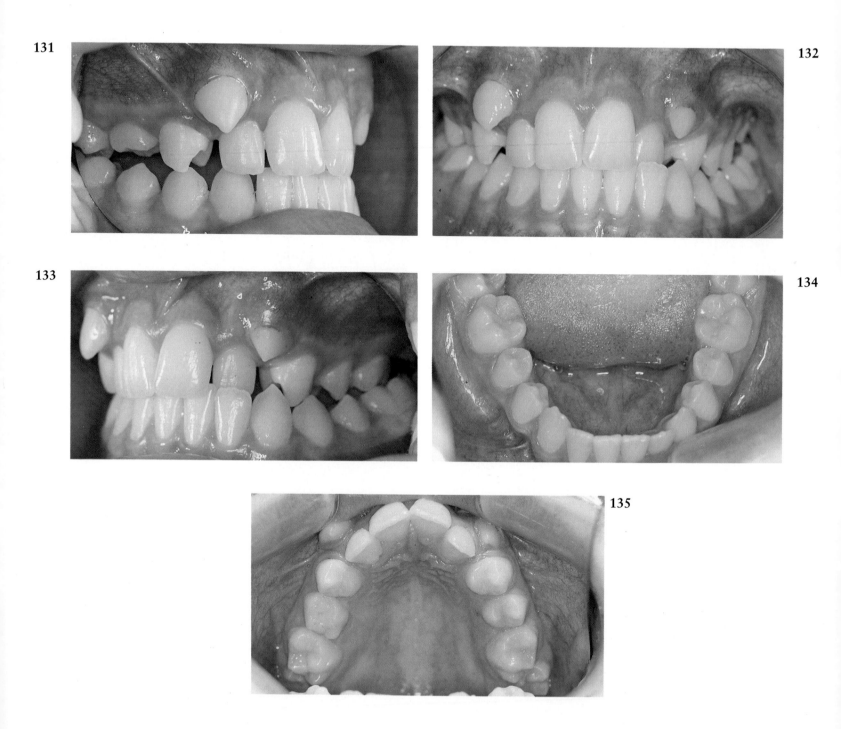

131–135 Many patients have maxillary and mandibular bone types which are much narrower than the 'non-orthodontic normals' had. The authors prefer to use zero torque canine brackets when treating such cases.

Missing upper lateral incisor result

If lateral incisors are missing and it has been decided to close the space, good torque control of upper canines is needed. Brackets to the dimension of the non-orthodontic normals may be used, but turned through 180°, to change the torque from –7° to +7° (136). This helps to move the canine roots palatally. It is helpful to engage in full discussion with the patient and family dentist before deciding to move a canine into contact with a central incisor. There is normally a color difference between the canine and the central incisor.

If the canine root is torqued palatally there is generally an improved appearance (137). Also, one could anticipate that a palatally positioned canine root will reduce the risk of elongation of the clinical crown later in life.

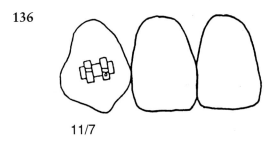

11/7

136 The upper right lateral incisor is absent in the drawing, and treatment included closure of the space, moving the canine mesially. This standard canine bracket has been turned through 180° to give +7°, instead of –7°, of torque.

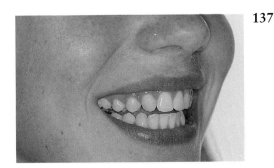

137 It is possible to achieve quite pleasing esthetics with canines in contact with central incisors.

Instanding upper lateral incisors

These teeth have special torque needs during finishing and detailing. It may be helpful to place a bracket rotated through 180° to give –10° torque (138). As a general technique point, it is important not to attempt to move such lateral incisors labially until enough space is available, otherwise they tend to pivot at the gingival margin. This makes eventual torque needs greater (139).

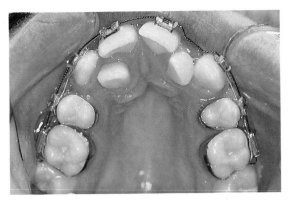

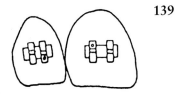

139 The upper right lateral incisor bracket has been turned through 180° to give –10° torque.

138 Occlusal view of instanding lateral incisors. Such teeth require special care with torque control.

Minitwin brackets

These are smaller versions of the normal twin brackets, having a rhomboidal shape. They provide slightly reduced control in return for the smaller size, and may be considered more esthetic and easier to clean (**140, 141**). Minitwin® brackets may help oral hygiene in cases with small clinical crowns or gingival problems, and they are available for incisors in the same specifications as recommended in Chapter 3. Canine and premolar brackets are available in the same specifications.

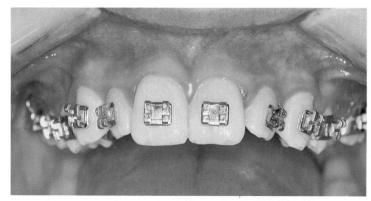

140 Normal Straight-Wire appliance.

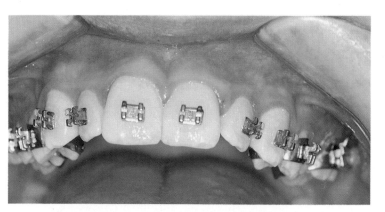

141 The same teeth with Minitwin brackets.

Patient Preference

Attract® brackets

This single wing system is much more comfortable than the twin bracket system, and it looks better. It is popular with patients and it is easier than twin brackets to keep clean. Such small brackets offer substantially reduced control, and can only be considered for cases which do not have particular rotational or torque needs. The case at the end of Chapter 6 shows the use of this bracket system on a bimaxillary proclination problem. The Attract® brackets are available in the same prescription as recommended in Chapter 3, for canines, premolars, and upper incisors. For lower incisors a 2° tip –1° torque bracket is available or else a Comfort® lower incisor bracket may be considered, having 2° tip and –5° torque (compared with 2° tip and –6° torque recommended in Chapter 3).

Starfire® brackets

Adults will often insist on the use of clear brackets, now that they are available, and these have excellent appearance when compared with stainless steel alternatives.

The bracket material is more brittle than steel, and the bonding method is based on silane, rather then the mechanical bonding which is used with the mesh pads on metal brackets. The brittleness and the different bonding method have caused orthodontists some difficulties in introducing the esthetic brackets, but these are gradually being overcome.

The esthetic brackets are used mainly on front teeth and therefore the recommended sliding mechanics and group movement works well, despite the increased bracket friction which theoretically can occur.

When using esthetic brackets, it is helpful to progress gradually from .018 round to .019/.025 rectangular steel, by using a gentle, more flexible wire after .018 round wire, and before a steel rectangular wire. This extra archwire can be .018/.025 nickel titanium, or else a braided rectangular wire.

Esthetic brackets are supplied with jigs which are helpful in achieving accurate positioning (**142**). Without jigs it was found that inaccuracies often occurred, due to the clarity of the bracket material as it came into contact with the tooth surface. Meticulous technique is needed, to minimize any excess bonding material, and a reduced etch time may be considered.

The authors are currently using special de-bonding pliers, with a rotational movement (**143**). Care needs to be taken to remove all excess bonding agent, and to place the jaws of the pliers exactly at the junction between the tooth and the bracket (**144**).

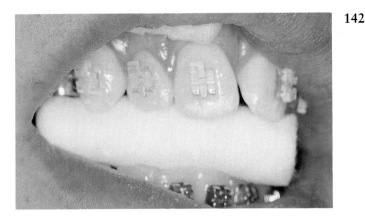

142 Esthetic brackets are supplied with colored jigs.

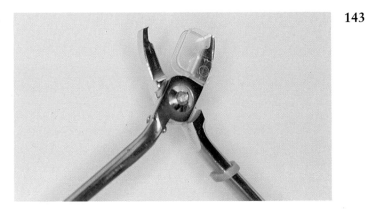

143 De-bonding pliers for Starfire® brackets.

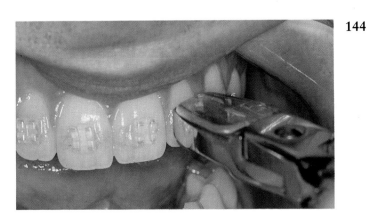

144 Debonding pliers in use.

5. CASE SET-UP

Bracket Positioning Concept

The placement of an orthodontic appliance is possibly the most important mechanical procedure in the treatment of an orthodontic patient. As the finishing stages are approached, proper placement of brackets can result in cases which begin to occlude quite satisfactorily with little effort, while improper bracket positions can result in cases which require several extra months of finishing and detailing. The additional time and effort that is required in the latter situation is important in a busy orthodontic practice. The only alternative to this unnecessary loss of time and effort is the removal of appliances before achieving the best possible result. This is sometimes done in the hope that the case will 'settle in' to a satisfactory position. At other times the tooth positioner is called upon to carry out tooth movements which are not realistic.

With the edgewise appliance, the most common method of determining the proper position for bracket placement involved measuring from the incisal or occlusal surface of each tooth. For example, upper incisor brackets were frequently placed 5 mm above the incisal edges of the teeth. When the patient's teeth were large, the bracket was placed more incisally compared with a patient with small teeth.

This variation in relative position on the tooth from patient to patient resulted in variations in the in-out position of the bracket, and in the amount of torque delivered by the bracket, because it was positioned at a different curvature on the tooth. A more reliable position is the *center of the clinical crown which is relatively the same in patients with large or small teeth*. Hence this position, as recommended by Andrews, was selected as the horizontal reference for bracket placement. The vertical long axis of the clinical crown was selected as the vertical reference line.

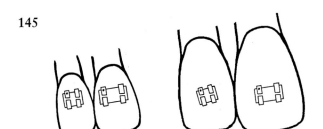

145 Brackets placed at the same mm distance from incisal edges onto teeth of different sizes. This gave different in/out and torque positions.

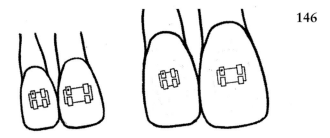

146 Using the center of the clinical crown provides for variation in bracket height depending on tooth size.

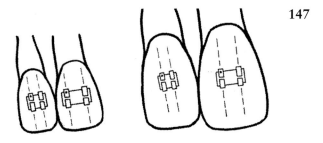

147 The appliance is crown related, and each bracket is placed with wings parallel to crown long axis.

Bracket Positioning Errors

Vertical errors

The placement of brackets too gingivally or incisally (=occlusally) is probably the most common general error in bracket placement. Often teeth are not fully erupted when appliances are placed. The orthodontist must visualize where the center of the clinical crown would be if the tooth were fully erupted. With experience, vertical inaccuracies of bracket placement can be minimized (148). It is actually surprising how accurate one can be at visualizing the center or mid-point of any given object, such as a tooth surface.

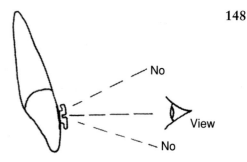

148 It is helpful to view the tooth surface from a horizontal aspect during bracket placement, and not from above or below. This will assist in avoiding vertical errors.

Rotational errors

Errors can arise from not accurately visualizing the vertical long axis of the clinical crown or from failure to evenly straddle this long axis with the tie wings of the bracket. It is important to key off the crown long axis of each tooth, particularly the incisors, and to *disregard the incisal edge*, in order to avoid rotational errors.

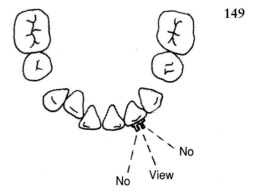

149 It is essential to visualize anterior teeth directly from the facial surface to reduce horizontal errors.

Horizontal errors

Because of the relative flatness of the facial surfaces of the incisors and molars, minor horizontal errors in bracket placement do not significantly affect these teeth. However, because the facial surfaces of the canines and premolars are curved, horizontal errors on these teeth should be avoided. For accurate bracket placement it is essential to visualize the teeth directly from the facial surface and also from the occlusal surface (149, 150).

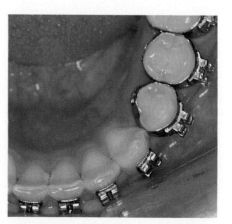

150 Canine and premolar brackets need to be checked occlusally with a mirror to prevent horizontal errors.

Avoiding Bracket Positioning Errors

Upper central incisors

Horizontal errors are normally not a major problem with the central incisors, because of their flat facial surfaces. There is a precise need to ensure that the central incisors are exactly the same length, and errors in vertical placement of the incisor brackets should be avoided. A common error involves placing these brackets too close to the incisal edge. Rotational errors can occur, leaving one or both incisors incorrectly tipped. This rotational error is frequently due to keying from the incisal edge rather than the vertical long axis of the crown.

In general, before bonding, it is important to contour bracket bases if they do not accurately fit the facial surface of a tooth. Also, it is necessary to avoid an excess of bonding agent under one area of the bracket base.

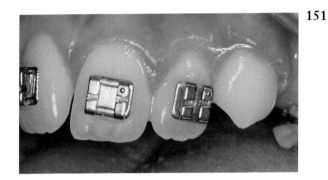

151

151 A correctly positioned upper left central incisor bracket. It is in the center of the clinical crown, with bracket wings parallel to the crown long axis. There is a need to avoid placing upper incisor brackets too incisally when new to the bracket system.

Upper lateral incisors

The most common vertical error is placing the bracket too close to the incisal edge. This leads to a lateral incisor that is short relative to the central incisor and cuspid. One reason for this error is that the lateral incisors are often poorly shaped and proportionately smaller than the central incisors. Hence, when the bracket is placed in the center of the clinical crown of such teeth, there is insufficient tooth structure between the center of the bracket and the incisal edge of the tooth, relative to the central incisor.

When this situation occurs, the bracket must be placed slightly more gingivally than the center of the clinical crown in order to allow for proper crown length. Rotational errors can frequently occur with the upper lateral incisor because there is often difficulty in visualizing the vertical long axis of lateral crowns due to their abnormal shape. Horizontal errors are infrequent unless the lateral incisor is rounded in its shape.

Upper canines

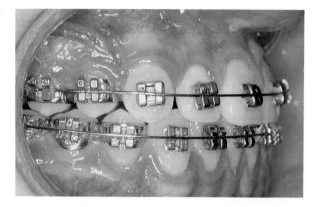

152 A correctly positioned upper right canine bracket. Canines are sometimes not fully erupted when the brackets are placed and the tendency is to place the bracket too incisally. Canine brackets should also be viewed from the incisal (occlusal) aspect to ensure horizontal accuracy. It is important to try to position these key brackets as accurately as possible.

Canines are sometimes not fully erupted and the tendency is to place the bracket too incisally. Horizontal errors occur more frequently with the canine teeth than with the incisors, due to their greater curvature. These may be avoided by checking from the occlusal surfaces of the teeth, using a mirror. Rotational errors in canine bracket placement can occur due to improper visualization of the vertical long axis of the crown.

Upper premolars

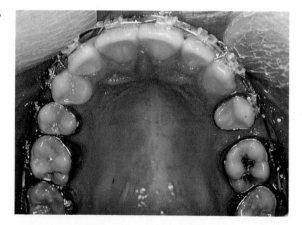

153 A correctly positioned upper first premolar bracket, viewed from the occlusal.

The premolars are often partly erupted and there is a tendency to place the brackets too occlusally. Horizontal errors are as frequent with the first and second premolars as with the canines, because they all have curvature of their facial surfaces. Rotational accuracy is generally quite good. However, in placing upper second premolar bands, an error can be made if the band is not seated adequately on the distal surface of the tooth.

Upper first molars

It is important to seek rotational accuracy when placing upper first molar bands. The buccal groove of the upper first molar serves as the vertical reference line on the facial surface of the crown and this buccal groove is normally angulated at 5° to the occlusal plane.

In order to position a 5° tip bracket correctly in relationship to this buccal groove, the band needs to be seated more on the mesial surface than on the distal surface. However, if a zero tip first molar bracket is used, as recommended in Chapter 3, it is possible to place the molar band parallel with the buccal cusps of the molar, and the band fits well in this position. The authors therefore favor a zero tip bracket.

The most common vertical error in first molar bracket placement involves placing the bracket too gingivally. This causes extrusion of the upper first molar relative to the first and second premolars. Horizontal accuracy is generally good, because of the flat facial surface of the tooth.

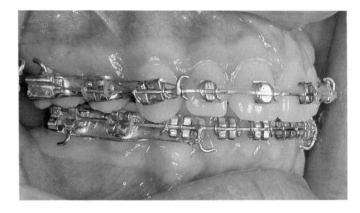

154 The authors prefer to use first and second molar brackets with zero tip, which allows the molar bands to be placed parallel with the cusps of the molars, where they fit very well..

155 A correctly positioned upper first molar band, viewed from the buccal. Horizontal accuracy is normally good, due to the relatively flat buccal surface of the tooth. The recommended upper first molar brackets have zero tip, and should be placed with the band parallel to the occlusal surface of the tooth. Equal enamel shows on mesial and distal cusps, or slightly more on the mesial cusp. There is a wedge on the lower canine, and there are upper and lower passive tiebacks, preventing space opening.

Lower incisors

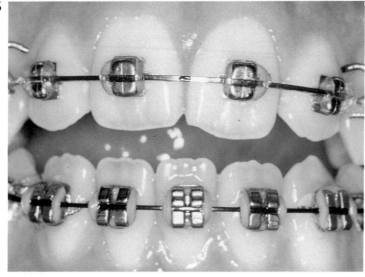

There is a tendency to place these brackets too close to the incisal edge. This results in a slight opening of the bite anteriorly during the finishing stages of treatment. Horizontal accuracy is normally good, due to the flatness of the facial surface of the lower incisor crowns. Rotational errors result in larger than normal inter-proximal spaces between the incisors in the gingival area. Such mistakes can be avoided by using the crown long axis as a reference point and not the incisal edge.

156 A correctly positioned lower left central incisor bracket.

Lower canines

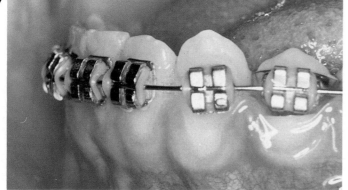

It is important to avoid the vertical error of placing the bracket too close to the incisal edge of the tooth. This leads to a slight open bite in the area of the canines during the finishing stages of treatment. Special care is needed with horizontal accuracy, because of the curvature of the facial surface of canines and bracket position should be checked from the occlusal. Rotational accuracy of lower canine bracket position is normally good.

157 A correctly positioned lower left canine bracket, viewed from the buccal, to confirm vertical and rotational accuracy. It is correct to key off the crown long axis.

Lower premolars

Sometimes the premolars are not fully erupted at the time of bracket placement, and hence the bracket is placed too occlusally. This in turn will lead to marginal ridge discrepancies between the premolars and the first molar. Accuracy in horizontal bracket positioning will avoid improper rotations of the premolars, due to their mesio-distal curvature, and bracket position should be checked from the occlusal. This is essential (**159**). Rotational errors cause marginal ridge discrepancies between adjacent teeth. This is particularly noticeable with the lower second premolar if the band is not seated adequately on the distal side of the tooth. This will lead to the most common marginal ridge discrepancy with the Straight-Wire® Appliance, which is the discrepancy between the lower second premolar and the lower first molar.

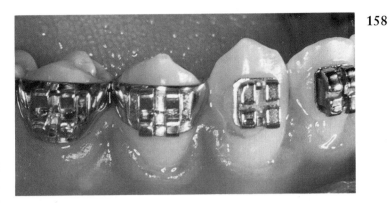

158 A correctly positioned lower first premolar bracket, viewed from the buccal, to confirm vertical and rotational accuracy. Premolars are generally banded rather than bonded in non-adults, for greater strength and accuracy.

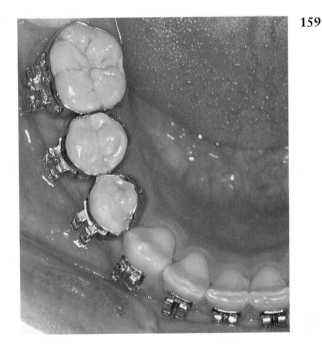

159 The correctly positioned lower first premolar bracket, viewed from the occlusal to confirm horizontal accuracy. Checking in this way is essential.

Lower first molars and lower second molars

Occlusal interference leads to the most common mistake with the lower first molar, which is to place the bracket too gingivally.

The most common rotational error that occurs with the lower first molar bracket is placing the bracket too far gingivally on the mesial and/or too far occlusally on the distal (**161**). Horizontal accuracy is generally good, because of the relatively flat facial surface of the tooth. After cementing molar bands, it is a kindness to the patient to turn in the hooks, to minimize discomfort (**162**).

The most common problem with lower second molar brackets is the vertical error of placing the bracket too close to the occlusal surface. Rotational and horizontal errors are not common with lower second molar bands.

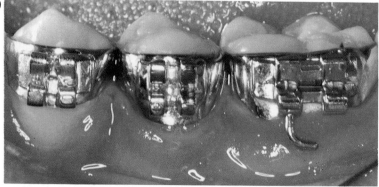

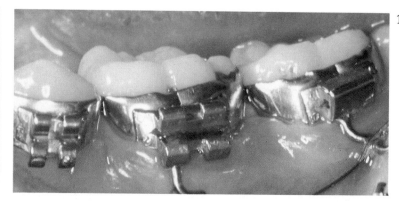

160 Correctly placed lower second premolar and first molar bands. It is important to avoid placing these relatively bulky brackets too gingivally. If biting sticks are used to seat molar and premolar bands, force should be applied to the bracket base, or the band material, but not to the bracket wing itself, to avoid damage.

161 Incorrectly placed lower first and second molar bands. There should be equal amounts of enamel visible from mesial and distal cusps. It is a common error to site the band too far gingivally at the mesial aspect of lower molars. Note the marginal ridge discrepancies.

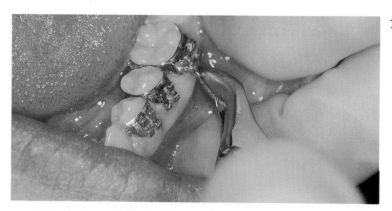

162 First and second molar hooks should be turned in after cementing the bands.

Upper second molars

The same rotational error in bracket placement occurred on the upper second molar as on the upper first molar, when using a 5° tip bracket, due to the fact that the buccal groove of the upper second molar is *also* angulated at 5° to the occlusal surface of the tooth. A zero degree bracket is therefore currently recommended. However, the most common error with upper second molar brackets involves placing the bracket too gingivally.

Separation

The authors have found that good separation of posterior contact points is essential for accurate band positioning in most cases. Elastic separating modules are normally used between molars, or molars and premolars, and are left in place for approximately seven days. Normal gray elastomeric modules may sometimes be used between small premolars, or between premolars and canines, for patient comfort.

Separation placement between upper first and second molars can sometimes be difficult, and the metal separators from TP (Ref 353–020) are often useful in this region. In non-extraction treatment, it is helpful to plan two separation visits. After initial separation, first molar and first premolar bands can be placed. Further separation is then placed for a week, before cementing second molar and second premolar bands (**163**). Generally, if elastic separators are left in place for more than a week, there is a greater risk of them falling out. If they are in place for less than a week, the teeth may be sensitive and difficult to work with.

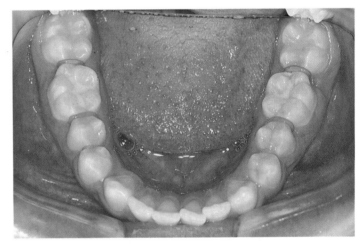

163

163 Elastic separating modules are normally left in place for approximately seven days. Normal gray ligation modules may sometimes be used between premolars, or between premolars and canines. Good separation is essential for accurate band positioning in most cases

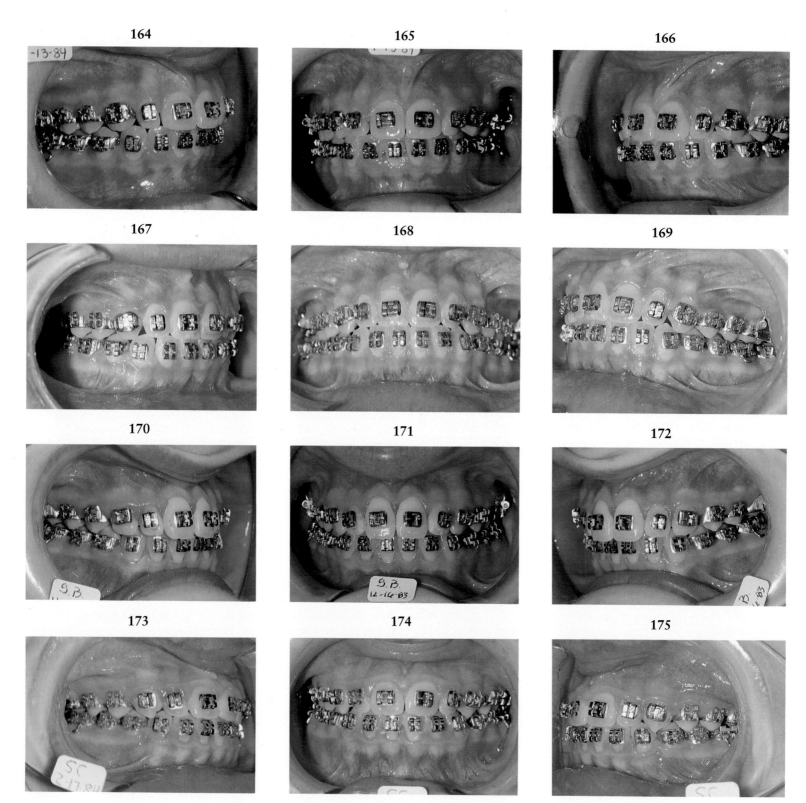

164–175 Examples of typical treated cases showing bracket and bond positions at the end of treatment.

6. THE TRANSITION FROM STANDARD EDGEWISE TO PREADJUSTED APPLIANCE SYSTEMS

Introduction

Prior to 1970 the Begg and edgewise appliances were the most commonly used appliances in orthodontics. These appliances had served the profession well for many years and quality results were achieved by those who devoted the time and effort to learn their proper use. In the 1950s both Begg and edgewise practitioners began to seriously consider ways to achieve the same or even higher quality results with less wire bending time and more simplified mechanics.[1] The result of this effort was the development of the concept of the ideal preadjusted or preangulated orthodontic appliance. Such an appliance was envisioned as follows: if an ideal gnathologic set up was completed on study models of a given patient, the ideal preadjusted appliance would:

- have bracket bases that accurately fit each tooth at a predetermined point, and
- have bracket slots that passively accepted a 'straight wire' co-ordinated to the patient's archform.

It was out of this concept that Lawrence F. Andrews developed the first commercially available Straight-Wire® Appliance. During the 1960s he collected 120 non-orthodontic normal study models (models of ideal cases that had never had orthodontic treatment) and described six characteristics or 'keys' that were consistently present in all 120 of these models.[2] Then, selecting the center of the clinical crowns as reference points, he measured the thickness, tip and torque of the clinical crowns of the teeth of each of these study models.

The averages or norms of this collective study served as the basis for the development of the Andrews standard Straight-Wire® Appliance.

This appliance became available to the orthodontist in the early 1970s. Shortly after its introduction, many other versions of a 'straight-wire appliance' became available and the effect of this development on the profession was most significant. By 1986 it was reported that preadjusted appliance systems in general were used more than twice as much as any other appliance system in the USA.[3] With this change came the possibility of, as well as the need for, a variety of changes in treatment mechanics. This chapter will discuss the most significant changes in mechanics that occurred in this transition from standard edgewise to preadjusted appliances, and how the authors modified and developed their technique with these appliances. While some changes did occur in the area of non-extraction treatment, the most significant changes occurred with extraction treatment and therefore a major emphasis will be placed in this area.

The mechanical treatment of most orthodontic cases can be divided into the following six stages:

- Anchorage control
- Leveling and aligning
- Overbite control
- Overjet reduction
- Space closure
- Finishing

These stages are not isolated from one another. They are sequential in order, and are integrated and overlapping with one another. Significant differences between standard edgewise mechanics and preadjusted appliance mechanics began to appear in each of these areas as clinical use of the appliances increased.

Anchorage Control

One of the first differences that became apparent was in the area of anchorage control. When archwires were placed on patients with preadjusted appliances, there was an increased tendency for the incisors and cuspids to tip forward as a result of the tip that was built into the anterior brackets (**176**). This tendency was greater in the upper arch than in the lower arch because of the greater amount of tip in the upper anterior brackets.

As a result of this forward tipping of anterior teeth, many orthodontists began to complain that these appliances 'burned anchorage' and some returned to the use of their more familiar standard edgewise approach. Andrews disagreed with this position concerning anchorage control.[4] First, he contended that most orthodontic cases were 20% undertreated relative to the non-orthodontic normal study models. This statement was based on a comparative evaluation of photographs of American Board cases with the non-orthodontic normal study models. Secondly, he proposed that if teeth were positioned according to the six keys on any given patient, the same amount of total anchorage control (or energy, as he termed it) would be required, no matter what fixed appliance system was used.

The authors tend to agree with Andrews' position.

However, while the total amount of anchorage control required for a case was the same with the preadjusted appliance system, the anchorage requirements at the beginning of the case were greater than with the standard edgewise appliance because of the tip on the anterior brackets. If these requirements were attended to at the beginning of the case and the crowns and roots of teeth were brought into their proper positions, then frequently the anchorage needs towards the end of the case were diminished.

As orthodontists began to appreciate this aspect of anchorage control with the new appliances, they took steps to manage their cases more carefully at the beginning of treatment. Some incorporated the edgewise principle of omega loop stops and molar tiebacks to control incisor and cuspid positions, while supporting upper molars with palatal bars and headgears and lower molars with lingual arches and indirectly with Class III elastics. Others preferred to use archwires without omega loops, choosing to bend the archwires immediately behind the most distally banded molars to control anterior tooth positions, and controlling molar positions with the same methods described above.

The authors chose this latter approach and found it worked well.

176

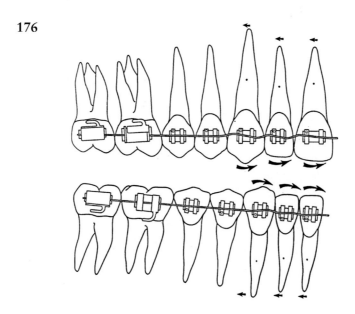

176 The effect of initial archwires on anterior teeth with preadjusted brackets. The tip built into the anterior brackets increased the tendency for anterior teeth to tip forward when the initial archwires were placed.

Leveling and Aligning

Two significant factors concerning leveling and aligning became apparent after preadjusted appliances had been in use for a period of time.

The first factor was the result of over-compensation during the management of the above described anchorage control problem. In an attempt to prevent anterior teeth from tipping forward during the initial stages of treatment, elastic forces such as elastic chains, elastic modules, and inter-arch and intra-arch elastics were frequently applied prematurely between the anterior and posterior teeth so that the anterior crowns were not simply held in position but actually tipped distally. This was not as significant a problem with non-extraction cases because the amount of tipping was normally limited by the presence of only minimal spacing or a lack of spacing in the arches.

However, with extraction cases, the problem was exaggerated because of the additional amount of space available for undesired tipping. The cuspids actually became the focus of attention in extraction cases because of the need to prevent their mesial tipping as well as the desire to begin retracting them into the extraction sites.

The premature application of elastic tension to these teeth caused them to tip distally, which in turn opened the bite in the premolar area and deepened the bite anteriorly (**177, 178**). This situation was normally correctable without adverse effects unless tipping was excessive. However, it did result in a longer stage of leveling and usually an extended treatment time.

The second factor concerning leveling and aligning was related to a desired compensation for the above described tipping, as well as a generalized awareness of a need for overcorrection during tooth movement and at the end of the case. With standard edgewise mechanics, compensation and overcorrection were handled by varying the amounts of first, second and third order bends in the archwires. The Tweed technique in particular was highly attentive to these needs for compensation and overcorrection.[5]

As stated earlier, the Andrews standard Straight-Wire® Appliance was based on the static tooth positions of ideal untreated cases and hence had no factors of compensation or overcorrection built into it. Proceeding with the concept of minimizing the need for archwire bends, Andrews introduced three new features to his appliance system.[6] He first developed two additional sets of incisor brackets with modified amounts of torque to be used on either extraction or non-extraction cases, as needed. Secondly, for extraction cases he developed a series of extraction brackets for the cuspids and posterior teeth to be selected according to the demands of the case. Thirdly, he provided hooks (which he referred to as power arms) to these extraction brackets so that forces could be applied closer to the center of rotation of each of the respective teeth.

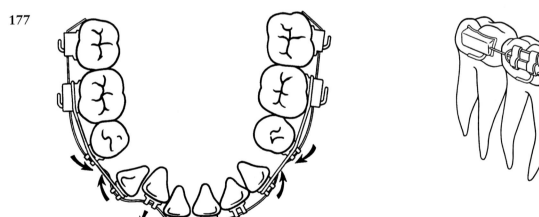
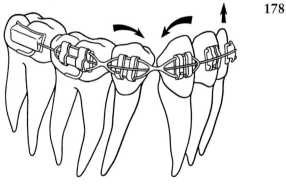

177 178

177, 178 Occlusal and right lateral diagrams of the lower arch to illustrate the effects of elastic forces applied to cuspids in the early stages of extraction treatment with light archwires in place (tipping into extraction sites, opening of the bite in the premolar region, and deepening of the bite anteriorly). Similar effects were observed in the upper arch.

Roth, who worked extensively with the appliance, saw a similar need for compensation and overcorrection, but did not wish to deal with the inventory concerns of multiple appliance prescriptions.[7] Based on his mechanics and treatment needs, he developed the Roth appliance, which he used and recommended for both extraction and non-extraction cases. It was not long before other preadjusted appliance systems were made available with a variety of angulation options. Thus the orthodontist was essentially able to choose an appliance for his treatment needs.

The authors evaluated the Andrews and Roth systems of brackets, as well as other preadjusted appliance systems. It was observed that no matter what system was used, if elastic forces were applied to the cuspids (even very light elastic forces) in the early leveling stages of extraction cases, adverse tipping occurred. This statement is not meant to be critical of any appliance system, but to point out this adverse tipping effect in general.

To help avoid this unwanted effect, the use of these elastic forces early in treatment was eliminated. In their place, figure eight .010 ligature wires (referred to as 'lacebacks') were placed from the most distally banded molar to the cuspids in each quadrant (**179**). They were used in any case, extraction or non-extraction, where forward tipping of cuspid crowns was not desired, but demonstrated their greatest advantage in extraction cases (**180**). In an attempt to minimize the forward movement of incisors, the archwires were also securely 'bent back' behind the most distally banded molars (**181**, facing page). The methods shown in diagrams **180** and **181** were not new to orthodontics by any means, having seen widespread application with various techniques. In addition to these techniques, molar anchorage was maintained with the previously described methods.

These lacebacks and bendbacks were used on a large number of cases. It was observed after a period of time that, despite the absence of elastic tension, the lacebacks not only prevented the cuspid crowns from tipping forward, but actually resulted in surprisingly effective distal cuspid movement without the tipping effect that occurred with elastic forces.

The figure eight ligature wires, when lightly and passively secured, initially caused a slight tipping of the cuspids with compression of the periodontal ligament in the area of the alveolar crest. However, because there was no continued elastic tension on these teeth, there was more than adequate 'rebound time' for the cuspid roots to upright into correct position as the main archwire took its effect.

179

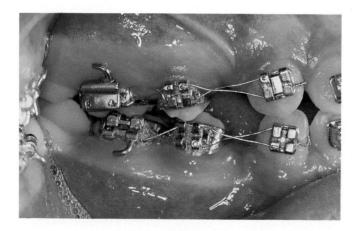

179 Lacebacks.

180

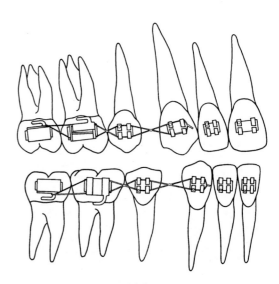

180 Use of figure eight .010 ligature wires (lacebacks) in extraction cases to hold cuspid crowns in position during leveling and aligning.

This theoretical explanation was supported by the clinical finding that when the patient returned for routine adjustments, the lacebacks were consistently found to be loose and to require minimal tightening. It is also possible that as the patient's tongue and food particles made contact with the lacebacks, additional minimal tipping occurred, but these were intermittent forces that still provided adequate rebound time for cuspid root uprighting.

It was observed that this technique allowed for approximately 6–7 mm of space opening in the anterior segments over a six month period of time, while leveling from light multi-strand wires into .020 round wires. At times this was more space than was desired (as, for example, with an

uncrowded bimaxillary protrusion case) and the lacebacks were discontinued before leveling was completed. If the case showed greater crowding than 6–7 mm, then the more crowded teeth were not bracketed and light push coil springs were placed in these areas to provide additional space opening (**183**, overleaf). These push coil springs were normally not applied until .016 or .018 round wires were in place. The forward tipping effect of these push coil springs was also supported with the above described anchorage control methods if necessary. In summary, then, the use of very light ligature wire lacebacks and primary arch wire bendbacks proved to be the keys to successful leveling and aligning procedures with the preadjusted appliance system.

181

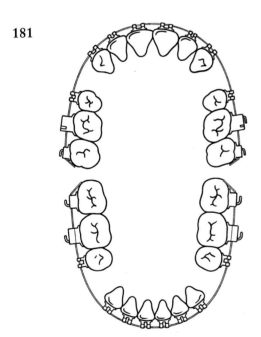

181 The use of 'bendbacks' behind the most distally banded molars to minimize the anterior tipping of incisors during leveling and aligning.

182

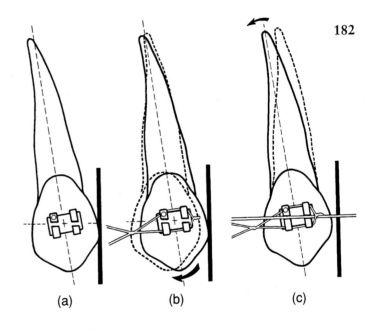

(a)   (b)   (c)

182 The effect of lacebacks on the cuspids. (a) Shows tooth after bracket was placed. (b) With the addition of a laceback, an immediate and very minimal distal tipping effect occurred. (c) Between visits a gradual uprighting effect occurred in response to archwire force.

183

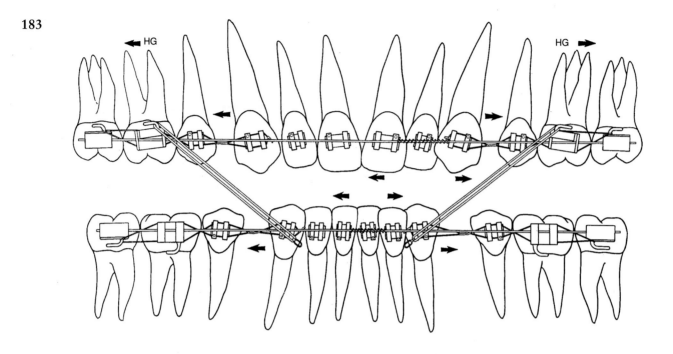

183 The supplemental use of push coil springs on more crowded cases. Note the blocked out lateral incisors with push coil springs in position. Also note the use of headgear, Class III elastics, lacebacks and bendbacks for anchorage support.

Overbite Control and Overjet Reduction

With the preadjusted appliance systems, the first difference that arose concerning overbite control was again a result of the tip placed into the cuspid brackets. Frequently cuspids erupted into a more upright position than was desired in the finished result. Therefore, when cuspid brackets were initially placed, the mesial aspect of the slot was more incisal than the distal aspect of the slot. As the initial archwires were placed in the cuspid slots, they then had to be extended gingivally to enter the incisor slots and subsequently created

an extrusive effect on the incisors which in turn caused deepening of the overbite (**184,** facing page).

On the rare occasions when the cuspids were very upright or even distally inclined, the most effective way to manage this situation was to leave the incisor teeth unbracketed or unattached. Lacebacks were then applied to the cuspids while waiting for the cuspid roots to distalize and the cuspid slots to become more parallel to the occlusal plane (**185,** facing page).

184

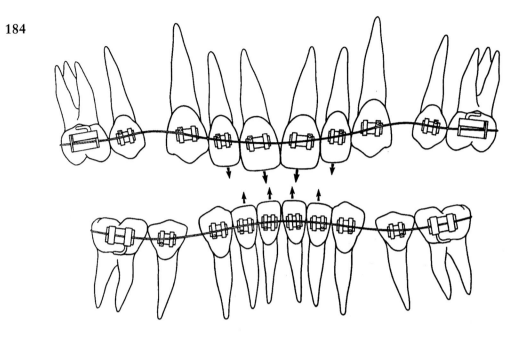

184 Effect of cuspid bracket tip on incisors when the cuspids were in a very upright or distally tipped position. Expression of the archwires caused extrusion of the incisors and undesirable bite deepening.

185

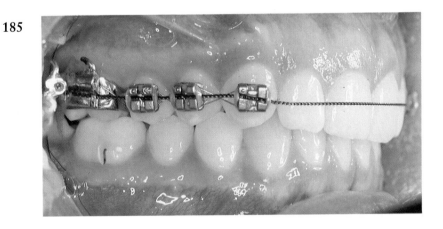

185 When the cuspids were very upright, or distally inclined, the most effective way to manage the situation was to delay placing brackets on the incisors. (If incisor brackets were already in place, then they were not attached to the archwire until canines were at a more favorable angulation.) It was also sometimes helpful to position the canine bracket with a rotational error at the start of treatment, and then reposition it ideally after a few months. In the case shown, the canine crown is distally inclined. Incisors have not been bracketed, and the canine bracket position has been varied.

The second difficulty concerning overbite control was actually a by-product of the elastic force effect discussed above under leveling and aligning. When elastic forces were placed against the cuspids during the early stages of treatment, the crowns of these teeth were tipped distally, causing the mesial aspect of the cuspid bracket slots to move incisally. This in turn caused the incisors to extrude and the overbite to deepen (see **177, 178**). This effect was not as great with non-extraction cases because the amount of space for distal tipping of the cuspids was frequently limited, as opposed to extraction cases. As mentioned previously, the use of lace-backs to the cuspids in the early stages of treatment prevented the distal tipping of these teeth and at the same time prevented the overbite from deepening.

The last factor relative to overbite control involved the importance of including the lower second molars into the system as early as possible during the stage of leveling and aligning. It was observed that complete bite opening was normally not possible until the lower second molars were banded and leveling had proceeded to the rectangular wire stage. This factor also applied to the standard edgewise appliance, but is mentioned because of its importance (**186**).

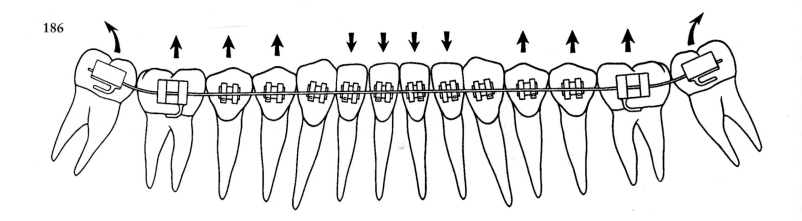

186 The advantages of including lower second molars in the system for overbite control.

Concerning overjet reduction, it was found that many of the principles used with the standard edgewise appliance were equally effective and applicable with preadjusted appliances. One difference between the two involved the previously described tendency for the upper and lower incisors to tip forward in the initial stages of treatment with preadjusted appliances. If not properly controlled, this created a need for more incisor retraction in the upper arch and hence a greater demand for anchorage control during this stage of treatment.

In the lower arch, uncontrolled forward tipping created a need to later upright these teeth when rectangular wires were in use. If this was not accomplished, the buccal segments remained in a slightly Class II position when the overjet was corrected (**187**).

A second difference between the two systems became apparent during the treatment of cases with severe overjet. With the preadjusted appliances there was a tendency to rely on the torque built into the incisor brackets to completely control torque during overjet correction. This control did not normally occur with severe overjet cases and upper incisors frequently finished in an upright position with inadequate torque, while lower incisors finished in a labially inclined position. This also left the buccal segments in a slightly Class II position (**187**). Of all of the factors built into preadjusted appliances, incisor torque was the least reliable in managing a large variety of cases. Frequently, third order bends were required in the incisor region of the archwires to control the torque.

The authors have found themselves 'adding torque' to rectangular wires in a high percentage of cases, seeking to achieve palatal root torque for the upper incisors and labial root torque for lower incisors. Changing upper bracket torque by 10° on the central incisors and 7° on the lateral incisors, and lower bracket torque by 5°, compared with the non-orthodontic normal values, reduces the amount of wire bending required.

Such brackets are recommended and are especially helpful in the management of starting overjets in excess of 10 mm, Class II division 2 malocclusions, and routine Class II treatment which is being treated to an end-result with a residual Class II dental base discrepancy.

187

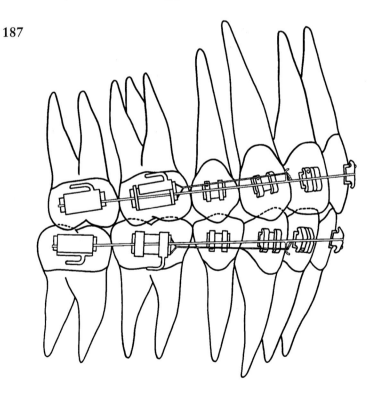

187 The effect of upright upper incisors and labially inclined lower incisors on buccal segments (a slightly Class II posterior relationship).

Space Closure

188

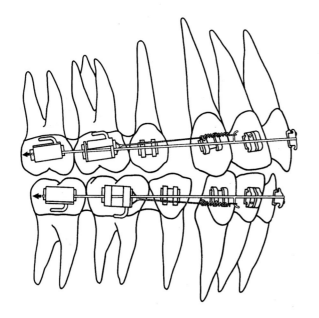

188 Closing loop arches utilized with the standard edgewise appliance for space closure.

189

189 Sliding mechanics on 'straight' archwires utilized with the preadjusted appliance system.

The most significant difference between standard edgewise mechanics and mechanics with preadjusted appliances was observed in the stage of space closure. This fact obviously had a greater impact with extraction cases but also applied to non-extraction cases with spacing in the arches. With the standard edgewise appliance, rectangular archwires did not effectively slide through the posterior bracket slots when the patient was out of the office because of the need for and presence of first, second and third order bends in the archwires. The orthodontist therefore normally used 'closing loop arches' which were activated in the office by opening the closing loop and moving the archwire through the posterior bracket slots (**188**).

For the first time in orthodontics, because of the level bracket slot alignment provided by the new appliances, archwires could be more effectively moved through the posterior bracket slots when the patient was out of the office. As a result, many orthodontists discontinued the use of closing loops in their archwires and began using various forms of 'sliding mechanics' to close spaces. For example, hooks were frequently placed in the anterior section of 'straight' archwires and elastic or spring forces were tied to these hooks from one of the molar brackets (**189**). A comparison between the advantages and disadvantages of both techniques provides greater insight into their relative merits.

190

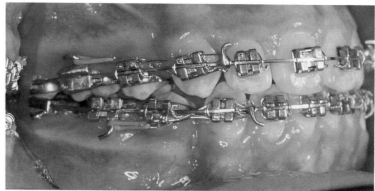

190 Sliding mechanics during the stage of space closure with preadjusted appliances.

Closing loop arches

Advantages of closing loop arches with the standard edgewise appliance:

- Precise control of the amount of loop activation (frequently closing loops were activated minimally [1 mm] which limited the amount of tipping that initially occurred).
- Adequate 'rebound time' for tooth uprighting (since activation was minimal and the closing loops closed rather quickly with minimal tooth tipping, there was ample time between visits for tooth uprighting and maintenance of arch leveling).

Disadvantage of closing loop arches with the standard edgewise appliance:

- Extra wire bending time.
- Poor sliding mechanics (the closing loop required activation in the office by the orthodontist).
- Tendency to run out of space for activation (after two or three activations the omega loop made contact with the molar bracket and the archwire needed to be adjusted or remade).
- High initial force levels.

Sliding mechanics

Advantages of sliding mechanics with 'straight' archwires and preadjusted appliances:

- Minimal wire bending time.
- More efficient sliding of archwires through posterior bracket slots.
- No running out of space for activation.

Disadvantages of sliding mechanics with 'straight' archwires and preadjusted appliances:

- Confusion concerning ideal force levels (since this was a new and untested system, there were no established guidelines concerning the amount of force to be used during space closure).
- Tendency to over activate elastic and spring forces which caused initial tipping and then inadequate rebound time for tooth uprighting (elastic and spring forces, while dissipating after initial activation, continued to create a tipping effect and did not allow for needed tooth uprighting).

In an attempt to maximize the advantages and minimize the disadvantages of sliding mechanics during space closure with the preadjusted appliance, the authors began reducing the force levels also during this stage of treatment. Instead of using springs or over-activated elastic forces (capable of generating forces of approximately 500 g) a single elastic module, of the type used to secure archwires to brackets, was attached to anterior archwire hooks with ligature wires extended forward from the molars (**191, 192**). These 'elastic tiebacks', when activated 2–3 mm generated approximately 100–150 g of force. Provided that the arches were properly levelled, this light force allowed for effective space closure

with minimal tipping of teeth and maintenance of arch leveling. When heavier forces were used, tipping of teeth occurred with subsequent binding of the archwires and delaying of efficient space closure. The use of .019/.025 rectangular wires with .022 archwire slots were found to be most effective, providing maximum rigidity while allowing adequate freedom for the archwires to slide through the posterior bracket slots.

It must be emphasized that effective space closure was by no means automatic with any method of sliding mechanics and that constant attention was required to prevent one of the following inhibiting factors from occurring.

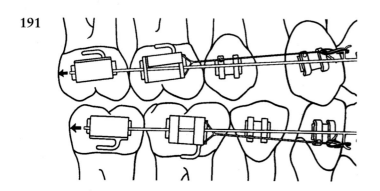

191 Illustration of the technique used during the stage of space closure with the preadjusted appliance system.

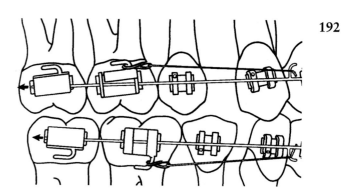

192 Modification of **191** with the elastic module attached to the first molar hook instead of the hook on the archwire. Both methods introduce light forces with effective space closure.

Inhibitors to Sliding Mechanics

- Inadequate leveling resulting in archwire binding.
- Posterior torque (torquing and sliding cannot occur simultaneously).
- Blockage of the distal end of the main archwire by a ligature wire.
- Damaged or crushed brackets that bind the main archwire.
- Soft tissue resistance (soft tissue build-up in extraction sites).
- Cortical plate resistance (narrowing of alveolar bone in extraction sites).

- Excessive force causing tipping and binding.
- Interferences from teeth on the opposing arch.
- Insufficient force.

In summary, while the use of preadjusted appliance sliding mechanics improved the efficiency of treatment in most cases, careful attention was required by the orthodontist to minimize these inhibitory factors. Very occasionally it proved necessary to return to closing loop arches.

Finishing

The real value of preadjusted appliances became most apparent in the stage of finishing, and the more accurate the appliance, the less time and effort was required during this stage of treatment. The factors of tip, torque and in-out compensation (including rotation control on the upper molars) allowed the orthodontist to spend less time treating the appliance with customary first, second and third order bends, and more time attending to the specific tooth alignment needs of the patient.

However, the misconception arose that no wire bending was required with the new preadjusted appliances. While very little wire bending was required in the first five stages of treatment described above, during finishing a certain amount of wire bending was required with nearly every case.

Firstly, it must be re-emphasized that all of these appliances were based on averages or norms and as a result they could not possibly meet the needs of all of the variations that existed in terms of tooth size and shape. While this was not a major problem since patients teeth were surprisingly similar, it did require that detailing bends be placed in the finishing wires of some patients to compensate for this variation.

Secondly, since bracket placement was a very exacting requirement of preadjusted appliances, when brackets were positioned improperly it was necessary to either reposition the brackets or place compensating bends in the archwires. It soon became apparent that it was far more efficient to reposition brackets at strategic times during treatment (such as when including previously unerupted teeth) than placing compensating bends during the finishing stages of treatment. Such bends could not simply be made in a single plane in space, but needed to be three dimensional, including the first, second and third order movements. This took an unrealistic amount of time and talent as opposed to repositioning.

Finally, the need for overcorrection brought about a requirement for archwire bending in the finishing stage of treatment. The authors found it better to use a single appliance system, with only a few optional brackets, rather than stocking a large variety of appliance prescriptions and then selecting particular brackets to meet the overcorrection needs of a given case. They found that there was not sufficient time saving achieved by keeping a large inventory of bracket systems, because of the variables concerning the distances that teeth needed to be moved, as well as the force levels used to achieve these movements. Also, it was found that the light force levels being used created much less of a need for overcorrection.

The following five areas of overcorrection needed to be attended to during the finishing stages of treatment of some cases:

- Tip control. Very little tip adjustment was required in the majority of cases. However, if, for example, a first molar was missing, accompanied by a mesially inclined second molar, then a tip back bend was beneficial in uprighting the second molar.
- Torque control. Torque adjustment of the upper and lower incisors was the most frequently needed compensation bend irrespective of the type of appliance prescription used. This was due to the wide variation in beginning incisor position, in the distance these teeth needed to be moved, and in the desired finishing position. Torque adjustment was also necessary in the posterior segments, particularly for lower second molars that tended to tip lingually, and for upper first and second molars that required additional buccal root torque.
- Archwidth adjustment. While standardized archform worked adequately for the majority of patients, occasionally the archform needed to be adjusted to compensate for disharmonies in archwidth. The most common disharmony was the narrow maxillary arch relative to the mandibular arch, requiring widening of the upper archwire.
- Rotation control. Most unwanted rotations could be controlled with rubber rotation wedges, Steiner rotation wedges and lingual elastics, without the need for finishing archwire bends. The exception to this was the rotation of upper and lower first molars. Since leveling and space closure mechanics were carried out by utilizing ligature ties to upper and lower first molars, these teeth occasionally rotated mesio-lingually. This was managed with the use of an offset mesial to the affected first molar.
- Curve of Spee correction. If the upper and lower arches had not been completely levelled by this stage of treatment (usually the result of too much force during a previous stage of treatment) then bite opening curves were selectively placed in the archwires.

Summary of Key Points

This chapter has presented a discussion of the most significant differences between the mechanics of the standard edgewise appliance and preadjusted appliance systems, and how the authors modified and developed their technique to best utilize these preadjusted appliances. The most important points can be summarized as follows:

- Because of the tendency for upper and lower anterior teeth to tip mesially in the initial stages of treatment with preadjusted appliances, .010 ligature wire 'lacebacks' extended from first or second molars to cuspids prevented these teeth from tipping mesially and served to distallize them effectively without distal tipping. The use of 'bendbacks' behind the most distally banded molar serves to minimize the labial tipping of incisors.

- The prevention of the mesial tipping of anterior teeth by the methods described creates a need to carefully control molar anchorage during the initial stage of treatment. The use of headgears, palatal bars, lingual arches and Class III elastics are most beneficial in accomplishing this.

- The mechanics developed to manage anchorage control and leveling also prove to be most beneficial in initiating overbite control. The including of second molars in the system as early as possible during treatment is essential for proper bite opening.

- Space closure is most effectively handled by utilizing 'elastic tiebacks'. These consist of ligature wires tied from first molars to anterior archwire hooks with small elastic modules. These modules, when activated approximately 2 to 3 mm, generate 100 to 150 g of force.

- The value of preadjusted appliances is most evident in the finishing stages of treatment, in that the majority of tooth alignment has been accomplished by this stage. However, it is necessary to place bends in the archwires to compensate for variations in tooth shape and size, for improper bracket positioning and to compensate or overcorrect for various tooth movements.

An edited version of this chapter was published in the *Journal of Clinical Orthodontics* in March 1989, and a fuller version, in German, was published in *Orthodontie und Kieferorthopädie* in 1990, under the title 'Die Entwicklung der Standard-Edgewise-Apparatur zu einem vorgetorqueten und vorangulierten Bracketsystem'.

CASE REPORT MB

A bimaxillary protrusion case, treated by extraction of four second premolars

This girl aged 13 years and 11 months presented with a Class I skeletal and dental pattern. She showed protrusion of upper and lower incisors, which resulted in her lips being apart at rest. Plaque control was not good.

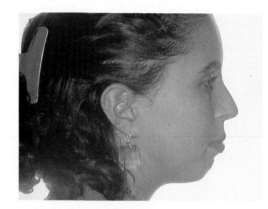

193

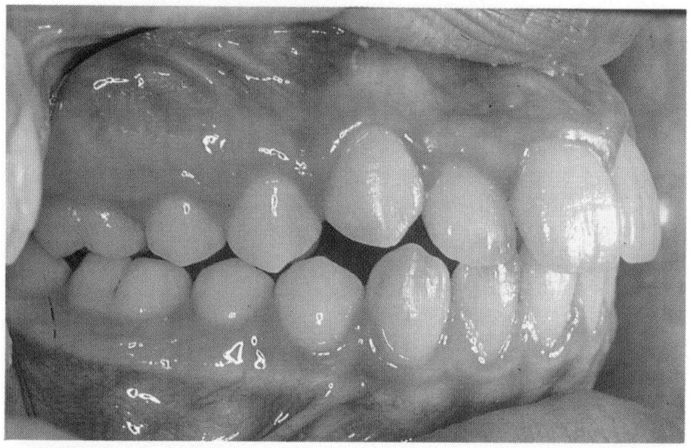

196

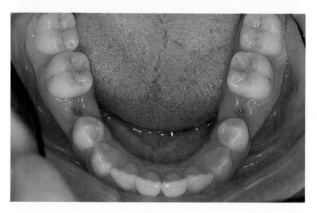

It was decided to extract four second premolars.

199

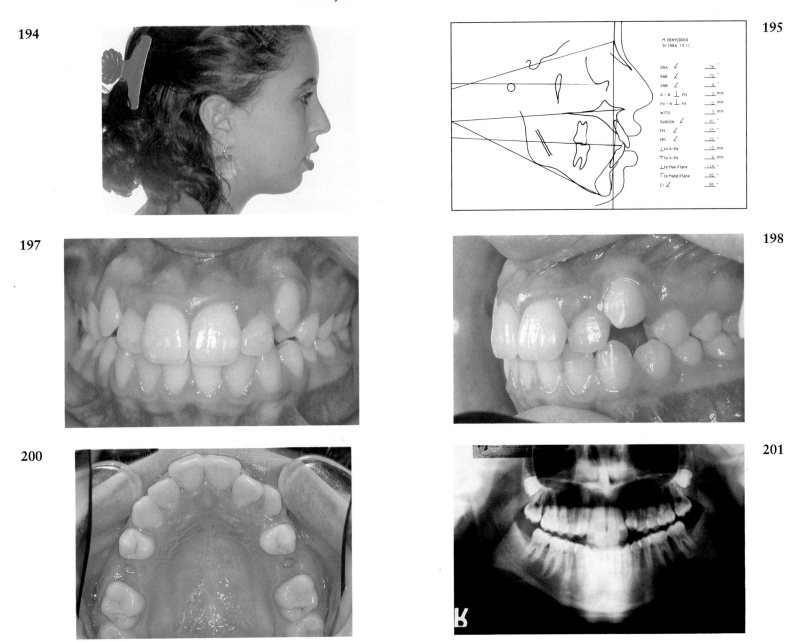

194

195

M. BENYEDDER
9/1984 13.11

SNA ∠	76	°
SNB ∠	72	°
ANB ∠	4	°
A – N ⊥ FH	1	mm
Po – N ⊥ FH	2	mm
WITS	1	mm
GoGnSN ∠	41	°
FM ∠	25	°
MM ∠	22	°
1 to A-Po	12	mm
1 to A-Po	9	mm
1 to Max Plane	114	°
1 to Mand Plane	95	°
CI ∠	86	°

197

198

200

201

Lacebacks and bendbacks were used, with .015 multistrand wires. Attract™ brackets were used to assist plaque control in this case, which did not have a need for correction of major tooth rotations. The upper left lateral incisor bracket was not fully engaged at the first visit, to keep force levels light.

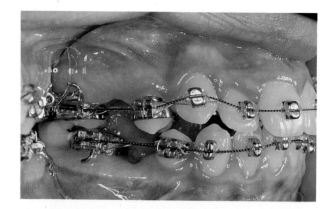

202

Lower leveling and aligning progressed more quickly than upper, predictably. Note the lower lacebacks tending to retract the canines away from the lateral incisors. This is not desirable, normally. The bendback distal to the upper left molar can be seen.

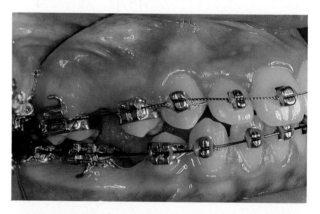

205

After three months a .014 upper round wire and a .018 lower round wire are in place. Lacebacks have been discontinued to avoid canine retraction. Bendbacks are placed in upper and lower wires.

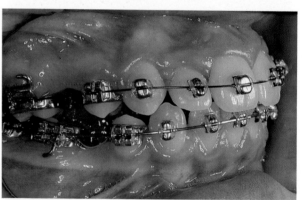

208

After five months of treatment. An upper .019/.025 rectangular wire has been placed with passive tiebacks. The lower .019/.025 rectangular wire has been in place for one month, so lower space closure can be started with active tiebacks using elastic modules.

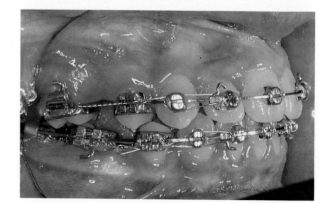

211

203

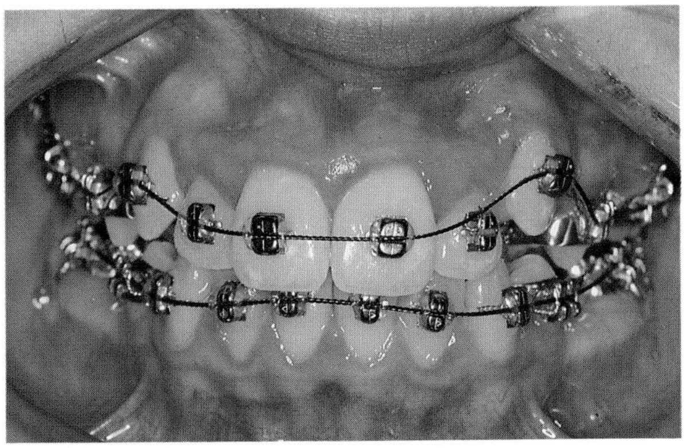

204

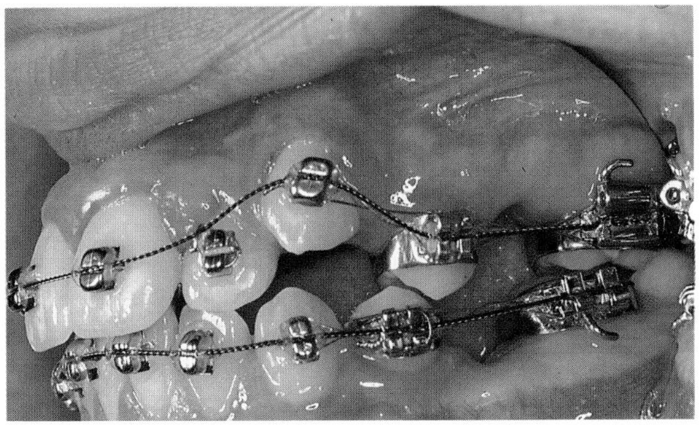

206

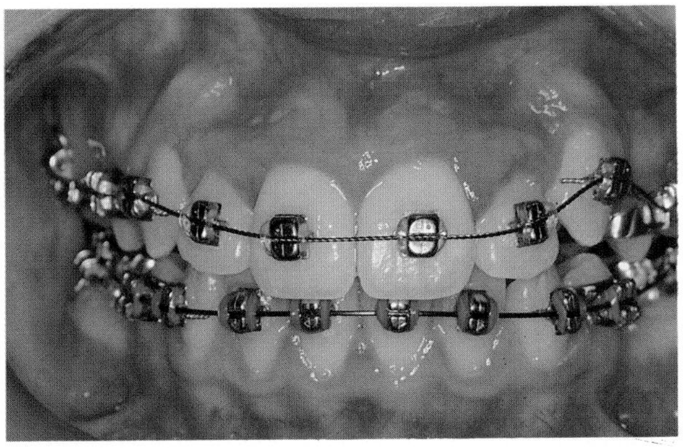

207

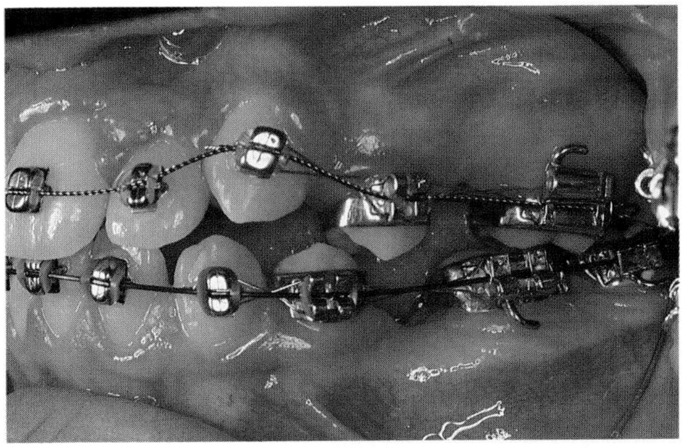

209

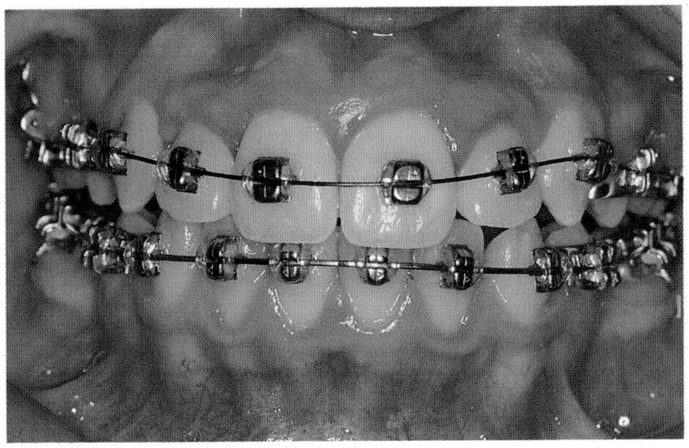

210

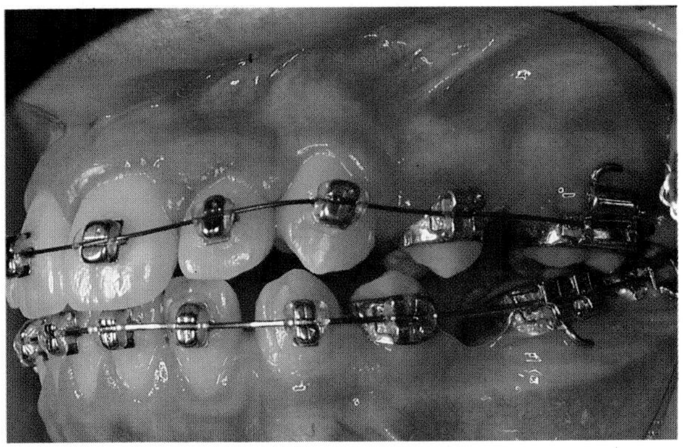

212

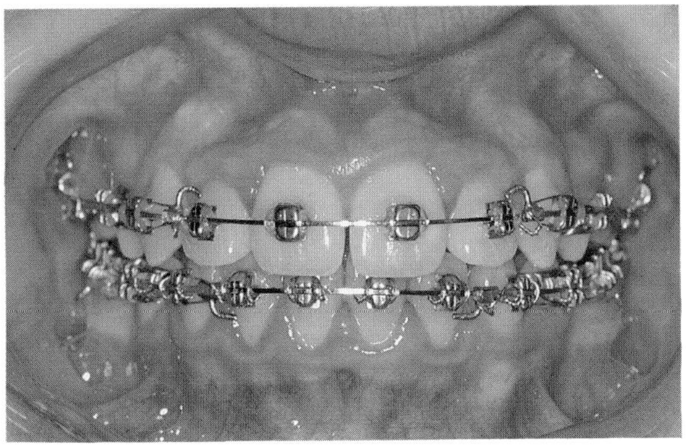

213

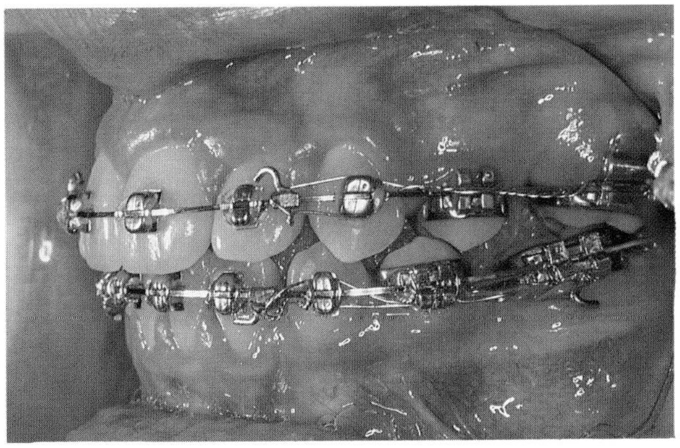

During space closure anchorage control measures can be used such as headgear, intermaxillary elastics, and palatal or lingual arches, as described in Chapter 10. Only intermaxillary Class II elastics were used in this treatment.

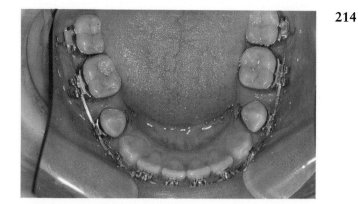

214

Active elastic tiebacks are being used for space closure, connected to upper first molars and lower second molars. The archwires carry crimped hooks, but the authors prefer soldered hooks.

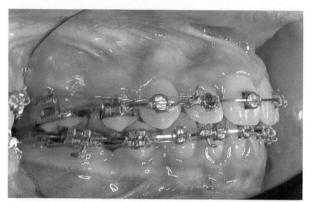

217

After one year of treatment spaces are almost closed. Brackets are tied with wire ligatures for control and full expression of the preadjustment features.

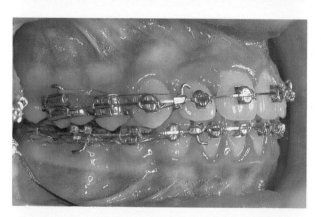

220

Archform has expressed itself. Note band and bracket positions. It was not necessary to band upper second molars in this case. Standard archform was used throughout treatment.

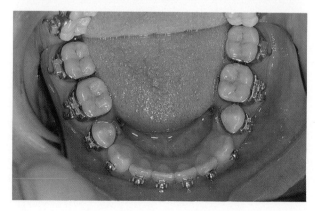

223

215

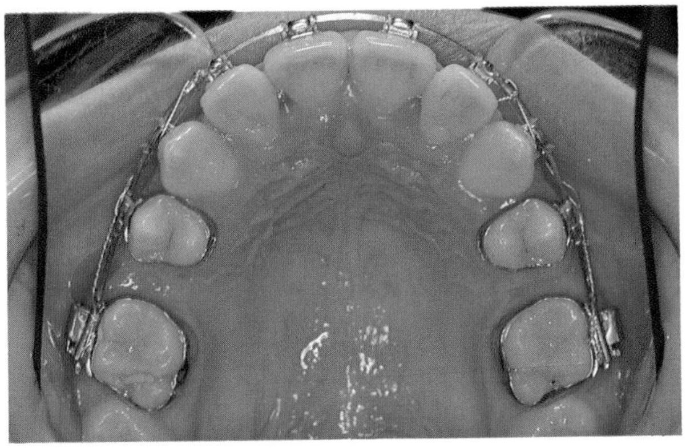

216

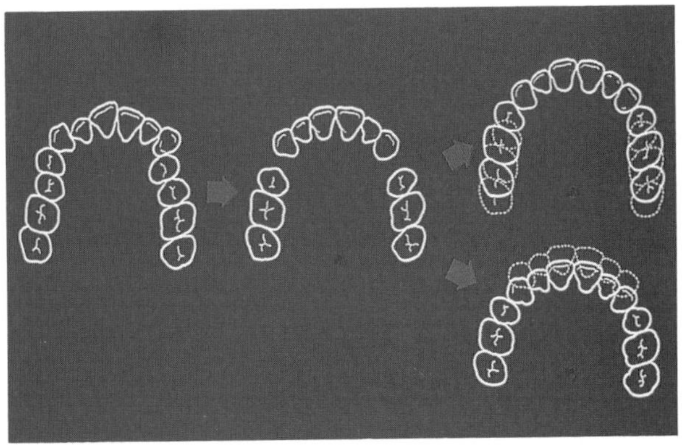

218

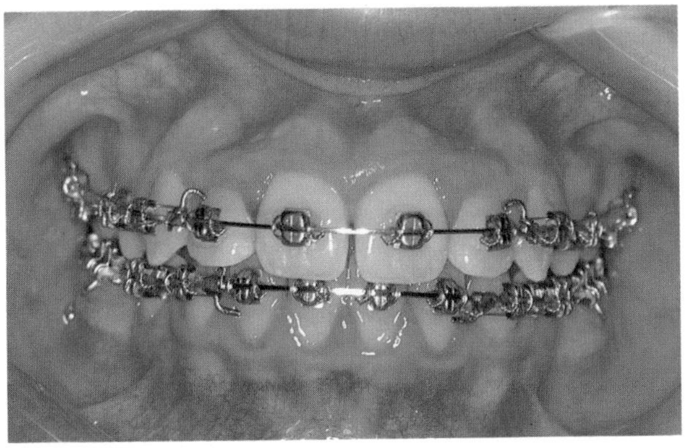

219

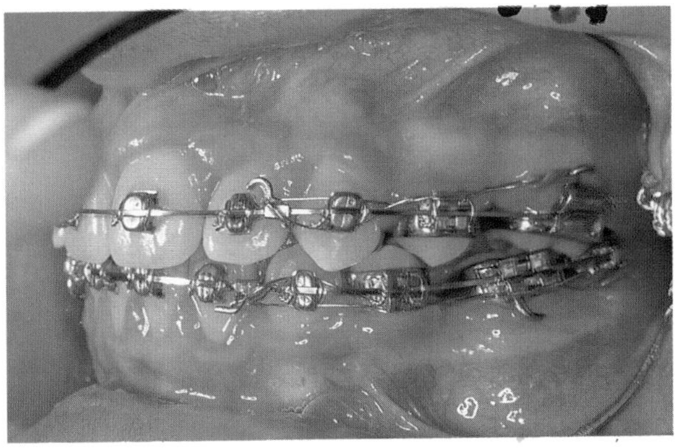

221

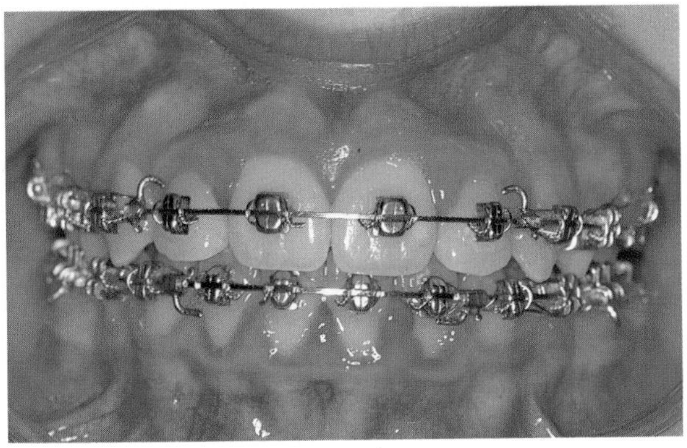

222

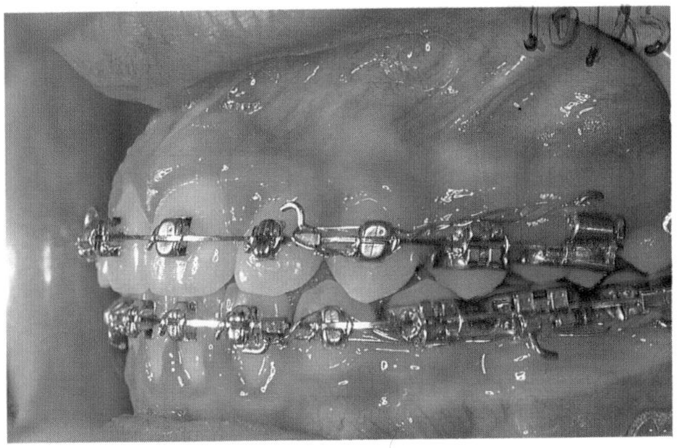

224

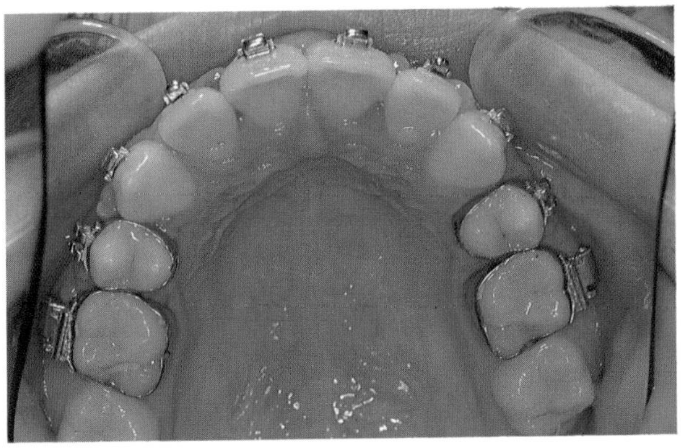

225

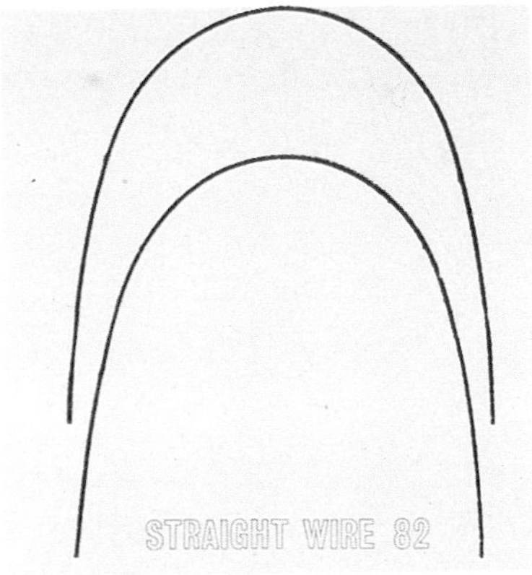

Rectangular wire can be seen protruding from the distal of the molar tubes, following the use of sliding mechanics. Intermaxillary elastics were used to control the overjet during space closure. Active treatment time was 18 months.

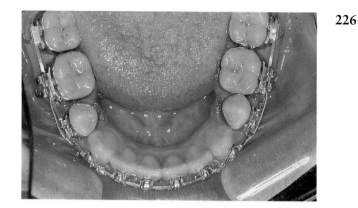

226

Upper and lower acrylic wraparound retainers were used at night for one year.

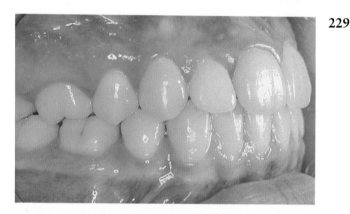

229

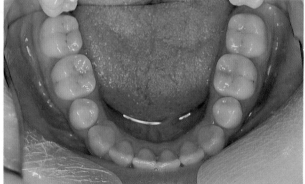

232

The case was treated as a minimal anchorage treatment, with no use of headgear, lingual arches, or palatal bars.

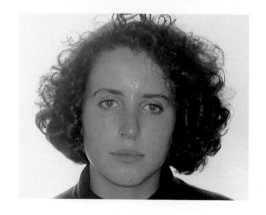

235

227

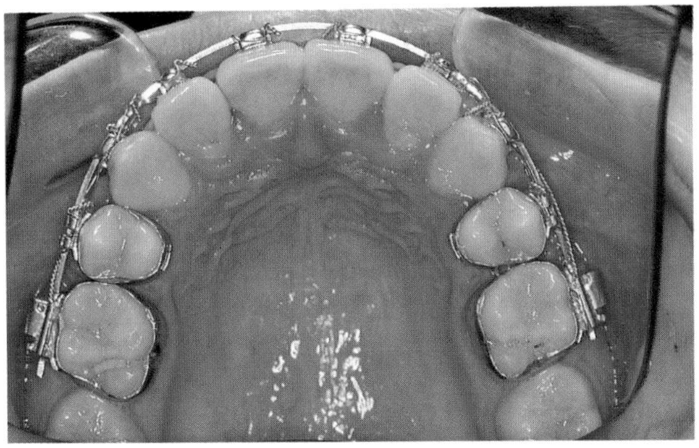

228

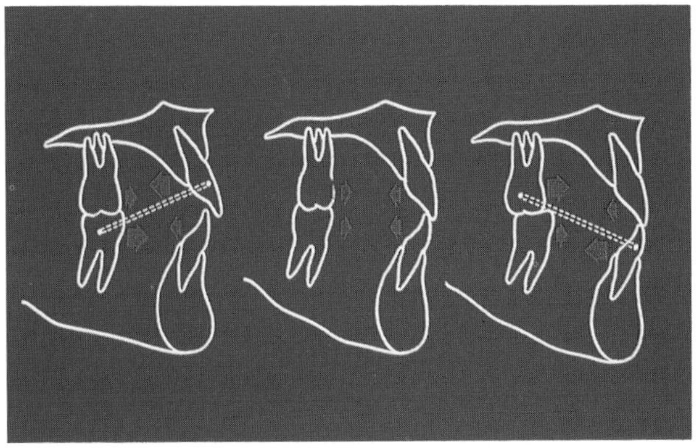

230

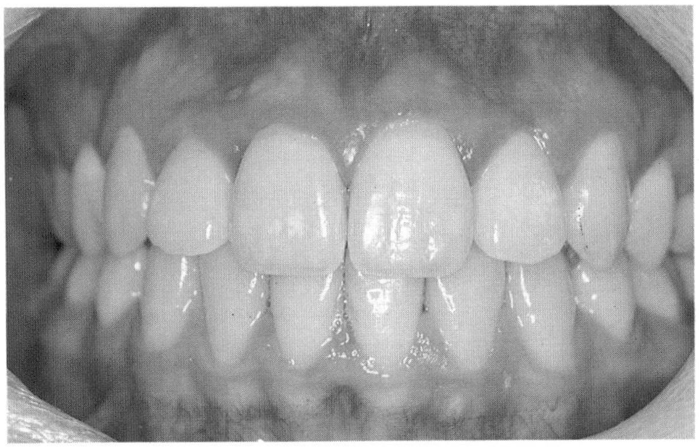

231

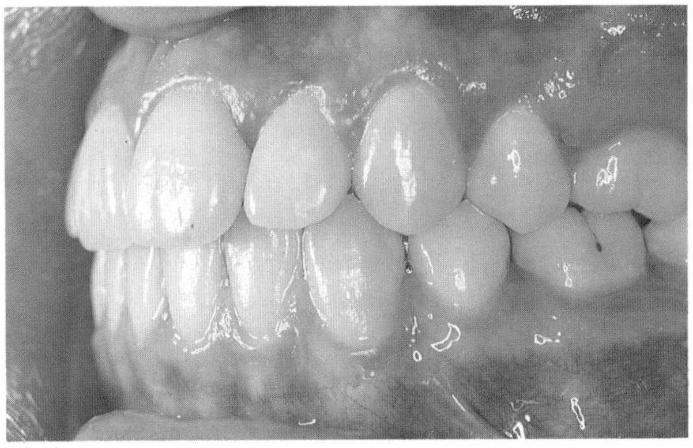

233

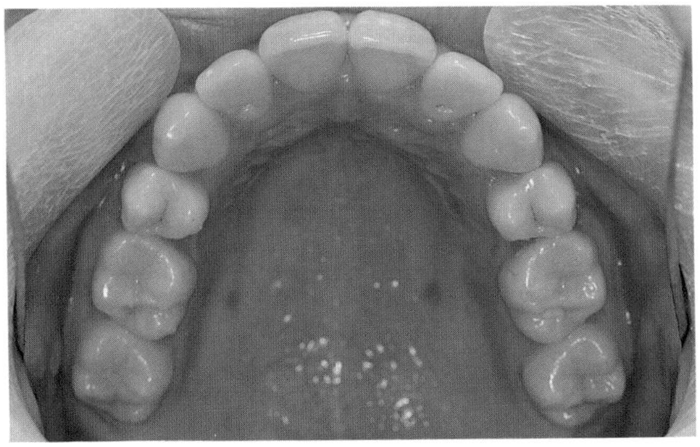

234

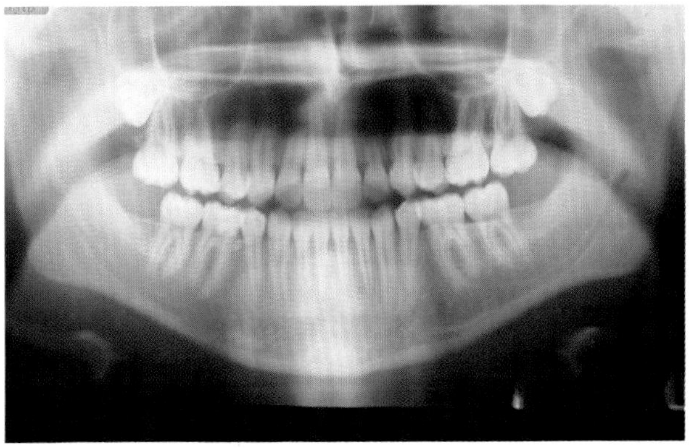

236

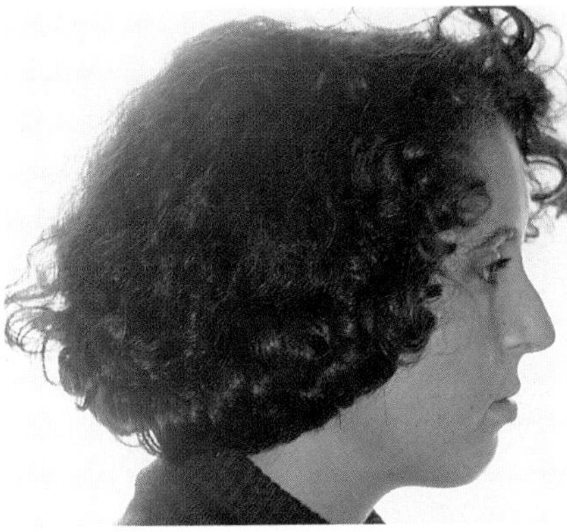

237

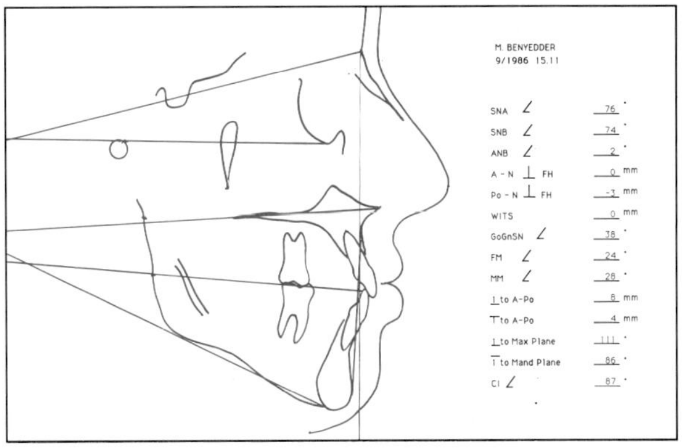

7. ANCHORAGE CONTROL DURING LEVELING AND ALIGNING

Leveling and Aligning

The transition from standard edgewise to the preadjusted appliance system has allowed orthodontists to treat patients more efficiently, with improvements in both the consistency and quality of results. Many techniques and procedures used with standard edgewise have been successfully transferred to preadjusted appliances. However, there remain significant differences between these systems which require specific variations in treatment mechanics and this chapter discusses methods of anchorage control which have proved effective during the stage of leveling and aligning.

Leveling and aligning is usually the fundamental objective of orthodontics during the initial phase of treatment. In most techniques, this stage is required before correction of major aspects of the malocclusion, such as overjet reduction or space closure. Although widely used, no definition has been offered for 'leveling and aligning', but in this text it will have the following meaning:

The tooth movements needed to achieve passive engagement of a plain, rectangular archwire of .019/.025 dimension, having standard archform, into a correctly placed preadjusted .022 bracket system.

Anchorage Control

Major tooth movements, supported by various methods of anchorage control, are accomplished *after* leveling and aligning is completed. However, *during* leveling and aligning, it is imperative that all tooth movements, even minor ones, be carried out with the final treatment goal in mind.

Clinicians have found that leveling and aligning produces certain unwanted tooth movements, and, if uncontrolled, the underlying malocclusion worsens, increasing the time and effort needed later in treatment, (for example, allowing over- jet to increase during the opening stages of Class II, division 1 treatment). Within this text the term 'anchorage control', during leveling and aligning, will have the following mean- ing:

The manoeuvres used to restrict undesirable changes during the opening phase of treatment, so that leveling and aligning is achieved without key features of the malocclusion becom- ing worse.

Long-term versus Short-term Objectives

It is helpful to consider leveling and aligning against a background of short-term and long-term treatment objectives:

• The short-term objectives, in the opening months of treatment, will be to achieve proper leveling and aligning into passive rectangular wire.
• The long-term objectives, to be achieved by the end of treatment, will be to achieve an ideal dentition, showing the six keys to normal occlusion, and with the dentition *properly positioned in the facial profile.*

Experience has repeatedly shown that attempts to rush the achievement of short-term objectives, by taking short cuts and using heavy forces, cause unwanted changes to take place. These make achievement of long-term objectives more time consuming and difficult.

238

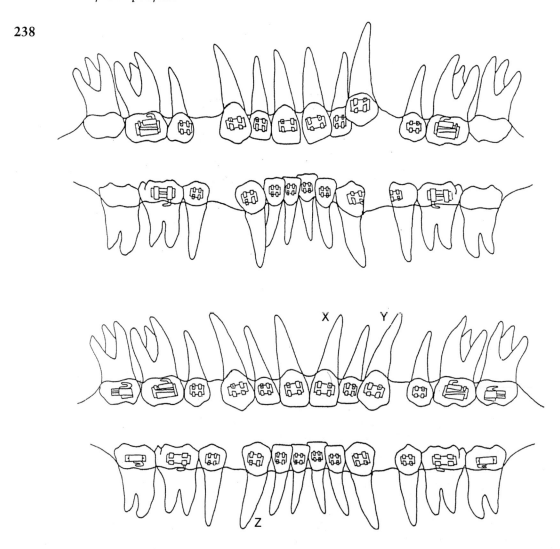

238 Typical tooth movements in early leveling and aligning with preadjusted appliances. There has been substantial root movement at X, Y and Z, which would not have occurred with standard edgewise brackets.

Control in Three Planes

Historically, anchorage control has involved limiting certain unwanted tooth movements while encouraging other movements, to ensure that the dentition is placed in an ideal position in the face at the end of treatment. It can be discussed in three planes: horizontally, vertically, and laterally. But it will be seen that the three are inter-connected, and failure to control one plane can cause problems with another.

Horizontally, anchorage control is used to achieve a correct antero-posterior position of the teeth in the profile at the end of treatment (239). It often involves limiting the mesial movement of posterior teeth while encouraging the distal movement of anterior teeth. For example, a 'maximum anchorage Class II division 1 case' refers to a treat-ment in which no forward movement of upper posterior segments is allowed, while preparing for maximum retraction of the upper anterior segments.

Vertically, anchorage control involves the need to try to influence vertical skeletal and dental development in the posterior segments (as with high angle cases), and at times attempt to limit vertical eruption of anterior segments, or even intrude these segments (240).

Laterally, anchorage control normally involves the maintenance of expansion procedures, primarily in the maxillary arch, and the avoidance of tipping and extrusion of the posterior teeth during any expansion phase (241).

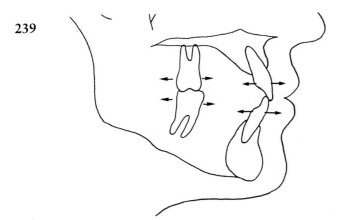

239

239 Horizontal anchorage control, early in treatment, assists later overjet correction, and helps to achieve a correct A/P position of the teeth in the profile at the end of treatment.

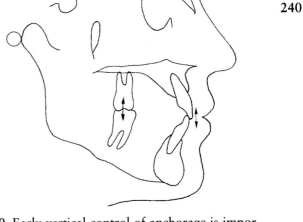

240

240 Early vertical control of anchorage is important, especially in high angle cases. Posterior vertical control of the molars can influence the height of the lower third of the face, at the end of treatment. If the molars extrude, the face height will tend to increase and pogonion will tend to move distally. Often this is undesirable. Anterior vertical control is helpful in early correction of overbite problems. It also helps to determine the occlusal plane in relation to the lip line at the end of treatment, which can be important in managing Class II division 2, and also the 'gummy smile' type of problem.

241

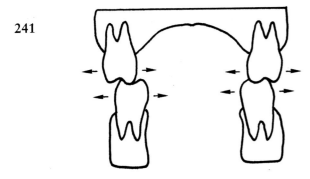

241 Laterally, anchorage control often involves the maintenance on changes achieved by expansion procedures. Bodily movement is preferable to tipping. Crossbites may be corrected in this way, if sufficient bone is available, and arch space may be gained, but there are limits. Muscle factors will cause relapse of indiscriminate expansion in most cases.

Anchorage in the Horizontal Plane

Control of the anterior segments

The first difference observed between the standard edgewise appliance and the preadjusted appliance system was the tendency for anterior teeth to incline forward during the initial phase of leveling and aligning. This resulted from the tip built into the anterior brackets and was greater in the upper arch, where more tip is built into the design (242–7).

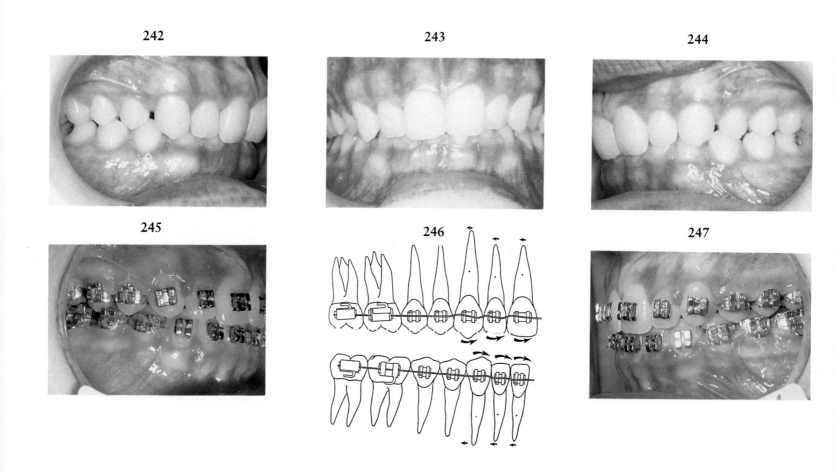

242   243   244

245   246   247

242–247 The effect of initial archwires on anterior teeth with preadjusted brackets: the tip built into anterior brackets increased the tendency of anterior teeth to tip forward.

Early attempts were made to eliminate or minimize this effect by connecting anterior segments to posterior segments, usually with elastic forces. But this created a greater demand for anchorage control during this initial stage of treatment. Also, if the elastic forces were greater than the leveling force of the archwire, there was a tendency for anterior teeth to tip and rotate distally, increasing the curve of Spee and deepening the bite. This was particularly evident in first premolar extraction cases, which will be the focus of discussion in this chapter (see **248–253**).

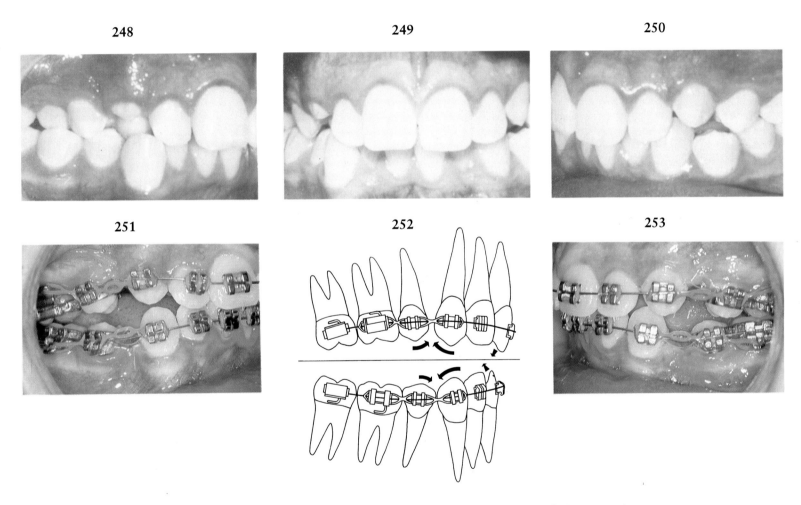

248–253 The effects of elastic forces, applied to canines early in extraction treatment with light archwires in place were found to be: (a) tipping and rotation into extraction sites; (b) bite opening in premolar regions; (c) bite deepening anteriorly.

There were two ways to minimize this effect. The route taken by Andrews[1] and later by Roth[2] was to maintain identical force levels and treatment mechanics, and to introduce features into the bracket systems to prevent unwanted changes. Extra torque was built into incisor brackets and anti-tip and anti-rotation features were put into canine, premolar and molar brackets. These were the 'extraction' or 'translation' series brackets, some of which were later grouped together to become the definitive Roth appliance. Power arms were added to some brackets to bring the forces closer to the center of resistance of each tooth.

The authors, however, took another route. This involved abandoning the traditional concepts concerning force levels and treatment mechanics, and re-evaluating the force delivery system to specifically optimize the performance of the new generation of brackets. However, this required time in contrast to the bracket modification alternative which could be carried out quickly.

A new system of force levels could only be developed by observing the effects of varying forces on numerous cases. Initially, minimum elastic forces were used, but it was observed that no matter what bracket system was used, there existed a tendency for anterior teeth to tip and rotate distally, and posterior teeth to tip and rotate mesially. Therefore, the use of elastic force was discontinued and lacebacks, extending from the most distally banded molars to the canines in all four quadrants, were introduced (**254–6**).

254

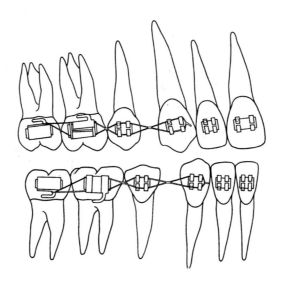

255

256

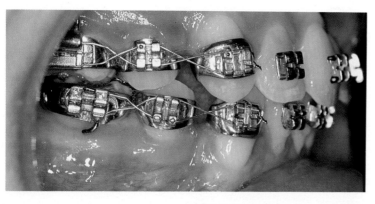
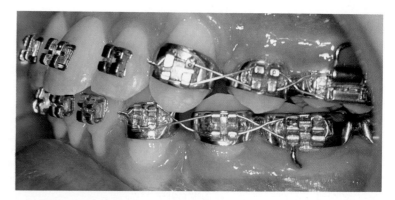

254–256 Lacebacks; .010 ligature wires used in an extraction case to prevent cuspid crowns tipping forwards during leveling and aligning.

The initial purpose of lacebacks was to prevent canines from tipping forward, but it was observed that, where necessary, these ligature wires were an effective method of distalizing the canines without causing unwanted tipping. The most probable mechanism of this movement involved the initial slight tipping of the canines against the alveolar crest at the gingival aspect of the canines, followed by a period of 'rebound', due to the leveling effect of the archwire during which the roots of the canines were allowed to move distally (257). With elastic forces, this rebound time did not occur due to the presence of a continuous tipping force, whereas with lacebacks, only a slight initial force was applied and not continued. Bending the archwire back immediately behind the most distally banded posterior tooth also served to minimize forward tipping of the incisors (258–260).

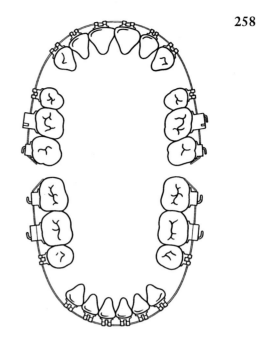

258

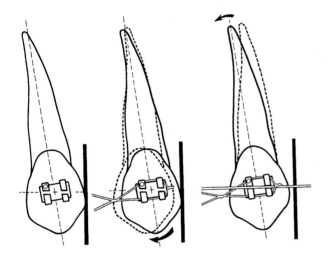

257

257 Effects of lacebacks on cuspids during leveling and aligning.

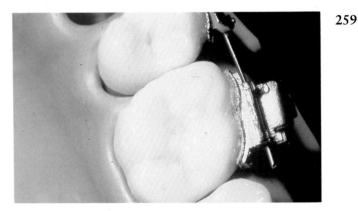

259

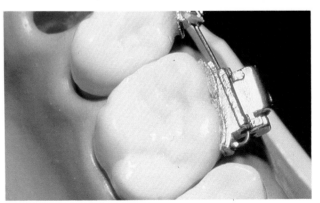

260

258–260 Bendbacks. Bent-back archwires behind the most distally banded molars, which help to control unwanted proclination of incisors.

In summary, the primary methods of anterior anchorage control during leveling and aligning for the anterior segments involved using lacebacks to minimize forward tipping of the canines, and to effectively retract them when indicated, along with bendbacks to minimize the forward tipping of the incisors.

Lacebacks consistently showed desirable clinical advantages, but no specific measurements were made by the authors to determine their exact effect. However, a study by Robinson in 1989 more accurately assessed their effectiveness.[3] He evaluated the lower arches of 57 extraction cases during the leveling and aligning stage of treatment. Approximately half of these cases were treated with lacebacks and half without lacebacks. The study showed that lower molars moved forward only 1.76 mm on average when lacebacks were used and 1.53 mm when no lacebacks were used. The lower incisors moved distally 1.0 mm on average when lacebacks were used and moved forward 1.47 mm on average when lacebacks were not used (261).

Therefore, there was little additional loss of anchorage in the lower posterior segments when lacebacks were used, but a substantial gain in anchorage in the anterior segments (approximately 2.5 mm per quadrant). In many routine cases, this created a situation in which no additional molar support was needed. Clinically, lacebacks were easy to use and were found to eliminate 6–7 mm of arch length discrepancy in the anterior segment without additional space gaining techniques or anchorage control. Cases requiring greater amounts of anchorage control are discussed later in this chapter.

261

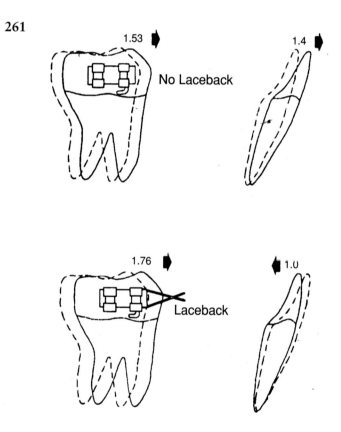

1.53 No Laceback   1.4

1.76 Laceback   1.0

261 In Robinson's no-laceback group, lower molars came forward 1.53 mm on average and lower incisors moved forward 1.47mm on average. In the laceback group, molars came forwards only slightly more than in the no-laceback group, 1.76 mm on average. However, lower incisors moved distally 1.0 mm on average, which indicated good anchorage support from the lacebacks.

Control of the posterior segments: upper arch

In certain cases, it may be necessary for posterior segments to be limited in their mesial movement, maintained in their position, or even distalized, to allow the anterior segments to be properly positioned in the face (239). Posterior anchorage control requirements are normally greater in the upper arch than in the lower arch due to five main factors:

- The upper anterior segment has larger teeth than the lower anterior segment.
- The upper anterior brackets have a greater amount of tip built into them than the lower anterior brackets.
- The upper incisors require more torque control and bodily movement than the lower incisors, which only require distal tipping or uprighting.
- The upper molars usually move mesially more readily than the lower molars.

- A typical caseload has more Class II type of malocclusions than Class III type.

Because of these factors, extra-oral force is normally the most effective way to provide posterior anchorage control in the upper arch; 262 illustrates the three primary types of facebow headgear and their force directions.

The authors favor a combination headgear (occipital pull and cervical pull) in most cases. The force levels used for the combination headgear are 150–250 g for the occipital pull and 100–150 g for the cervical pull. These force values allow for slightly stronger pull on the occipital component of the headgear, keeping forces directed slightly above the occlusal plane and minimizing the tendency for vertical extrusion of the upper posterior teeth, while simultaneously allowing effective distalization of the molar.

262

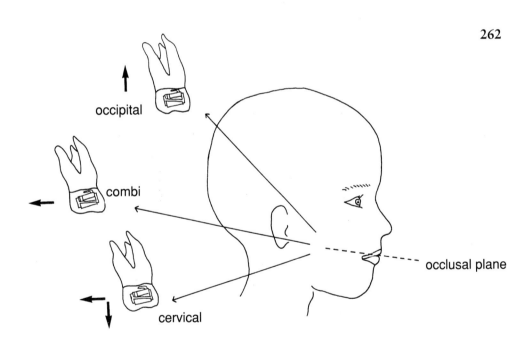

262 The three primary types of facebow headgears. The authors favor a combination type of headgear, with a direction of pull along or slightly above the occlusal plane.

263

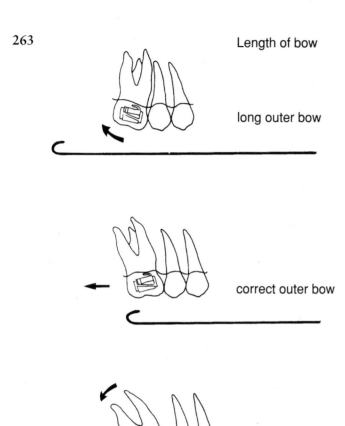

Length of bow

long outer bow

correct outer bow

short outer bow

The length of the outer bow of the headgear is important to avoid unwanted molar tipping. It should end adjacent to the upper first molar (263). An extended outer bow or an outer bow bent downward provides a greater tendency for distal tipping on the crown of the first molar, while using a shorter outer bow, or tipping up of the outer bow, causes a greater tendency for the roots to be distalized ahead of the crowns, as shown in the illustration. On high angle cases where little distalization of the molar is required, an occipital headgear alone can be utilized. In very low angle cases, where musculature is strong enough to minimize vertical extrusion of the posterior teeth, a cervical headgear alone can be considered.

A secondary method of anchorage support in the upper posterior segment is the palatal bar. This is normally placed when the upper molars have been properly rotated and are situated in a Class I relationship to the lower molars. The palatal bar can be constructed of heavy .045 or .051 inch (1.1 oer 1.3 mm) round wire extending from molar to molar with a loop placed in the middle of the palate and the wire about .25 inch (2 mm) from the roof of the palate (264). It is soldered to the molar bands.

263 Illustration of the correct length of the outer bow of the combination headgear. Forces are directed through the center of resistance of the molars, avoiding unwanted tipping.

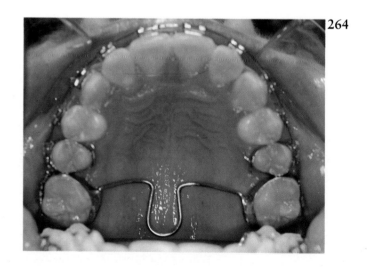

264

264 Fixed palatal bar situated approximately 2 mm from the roof of the palate.

Control of posterior segments: lower arch

When extra anchorage support is needed in the lower posterior segments, a lingual arch can be placed at the initial banding visit. The authors prefer a .045 or .051 soldered lingual arch with loops placed anterior to the molars. The lingual arch remains in position during leveling and aligning and is helpful during the initial phase of unraveling crowded incisors with lacebacks. The use of the lingual arch and lacebacks is adequate for anchorage support in 80–90% of all cases presenting for treatment.

In cases with severe anterior crowding, where more anchorage support is needed, push coil springs can be added in the areas of the crowded and blocked out incisors, and Class III elastics can be applied to the lower cuspids once the .016 round wire stage has been reached (265 below, and 267–275 overleaf).

The authors prefer to delay Class III elastics until at least the .016 round wire stage to prevent extrusion of the incisors. Figure 266 shows the force vectors that are generated during the use of Class III elastics. When the downward and forward vector of force on the upper molar is contraindicated, a palatal bar and high pull facebow headgear can be used to prevent this effect. The extrusive effect of Class III elastics on the lower incisors can be minimized by waiting until at least the .016 round wire stage so that the primary force vector becomes a distalizing force on the lower anterior segment.

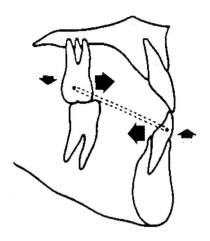

266

266 Force vectors which are introduced to the dentition when Class III elastics are used.

265

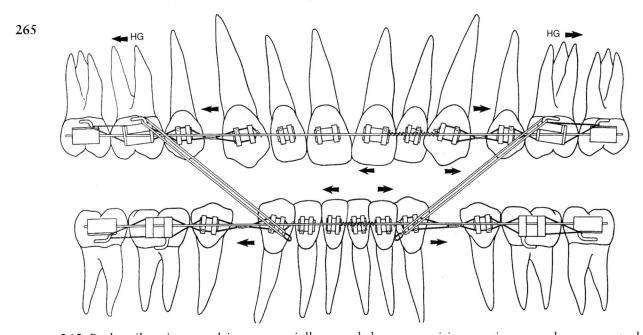

265 Push-coil springs used in an especially crowded case, requiring maximum anchorage control. Headgear, Class III elastics to Kobayashi hooks, lacebacks and bendback archwires are all used. See also 267–275 overleaf.

267 268 269

270 271 272

273 274 275

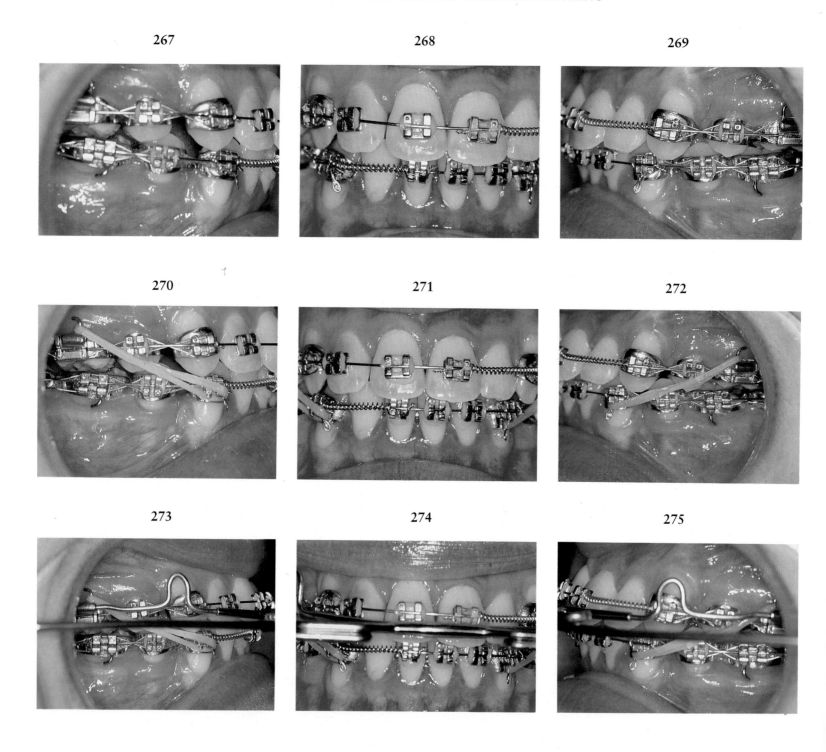

267–275 Push-coil springs used in an especially crowded case, requiring maximum anchorage control. Headgear, Class III elastics to Kobayashi hooks, lacebacks and bendback archwires are all used.

Anchorage Assessment in the Vertical Plane

There are two important areas of anchorage control in the vertical plane (see **240**):

- Incisor vertical control. Anterior control is needed in leveling and aligning of deep bite cases, to restrict temporary increases in the overbite.

- Molar vertical control. Molar and premolar control is needed in skeletal high-angle cases, to prevent extrusion of posterior teeth and further opening of the mandibular plane angle.

Incisor vertical control

Preadjusted appliances produce a transitional deepening of the anterior overbite during leveling and aligning, mainly due to the tip in the canine brackets. This effect is more extreme in the upper arch. If canines are tipped distally, the mesial aspect of the canine bracket slot is directed in an occlusal direction. As the archwire passes through the canine bracket slot, there is a tendency for it to lay incisal to the incisor bracket slots. If the wire is then engaged in the incisors, it causes extrusion of these teeth which is undesirable in many cases (**276**). This effect can be avoided either by not initially bracketing the incisors (see **286**) or by not tying the archwire into the incisor brackets, but allowing it to lay incisal to the brackets until the canine roots have been uprighted and moved distally under control of the lacebacks.

Once the canine roots have been distalized, the canine bracket slots will be more parallel to the occlusal plane and the incisors can be engaged without causing unwanted extrusion.

276

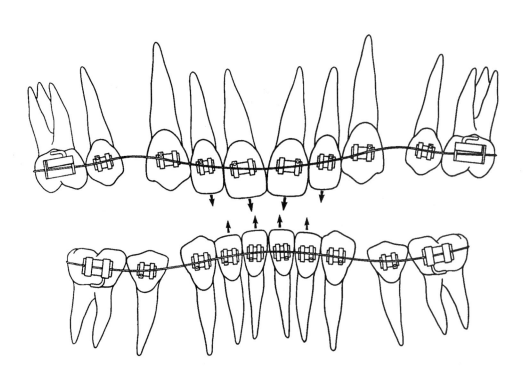

276 The effects of canine bracket tip. If canines are upright or distally inclined at the start of treatment, there can be resulting extrusion of the incisors, with undesirable bite deepening.

It is important to avoid early archwire engagement of high labial canines so that unwanted vertical movement of lateral incisors and premolars does not occur, and arch form is not significantly distorted during early phases of treatment with light wires (277–280).

On occasion, the authors will use intrusion arches (utility arches or base arches) for incisor intrusion. Since this procedure is used infrequently, it will not be discussed in detail in the text.

277

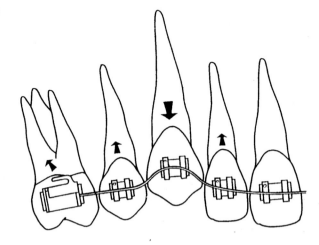

279

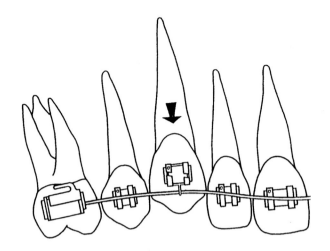

278

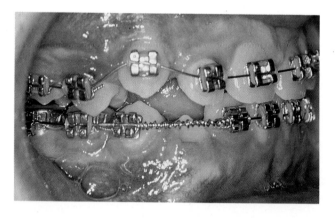

277–278 Excessive deflection of archwires into unerupted canines causes vertical movement of lateral incisors and premolars, and should be avoided.

280

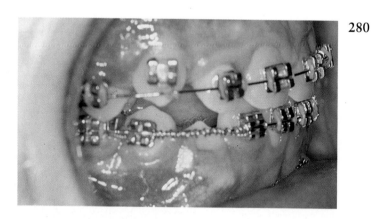

279–280 The unwanted effects in **277–278** may be minimized by lightly tying canines to the primary archwire with elastic thread, instead of fully engaging the archwire into the canine bracket slot.

Molar vertical control

The following methods of vertical molar control (see **240**) can be considered when treating higher angle cases:

- Upper second molars are generally not initially banded or bracketed, to minimize extrusion of these teeth. If they require banding, an archwire step can be placed behind the first molar to avoid extrusion.
- If the upper first molars require expansion, an attempt is made to achieve bodily movement rather than tipping, to avoid extrusion of the palatal cusps. This is best accomplished with a fixed expander, sometimes combined with a high-pull headgear.
- If palatal bars are used, they are designed to lie away from the palate by approximately 2 mm so that the tongue can exert a vertical intrusive effect on these teeth (**264, 281**).
- When headgears are used in high-angle cases, either a combination pull or a high-pull headgear is used. The cervical pull headgear is avoided.
- In some cases, an upper or lower posterior biteplate in the molar region is helpful to minimize extrusion of molars.

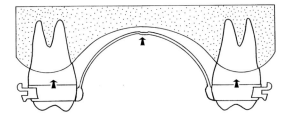

281 Palatal bars may be designed to lie away from the palate by approximately 2 mm, so that tongue forces can assist vertical control. See also **264** (p. 98).

Anchorage Assessment in the Lateral (Coronal) Plane

In most cases, no special care is needed to maintain lateral anchorage control, but the following points are important in certain treatments:

- *Intercanine Width.* Upper and lower inter-canine width should be kept as close as possible to starting dimensions for stability, and care should be taken to ensure that crowding is not relieved by uncontrolled expansion of the upper and lower arches.
- *Molar Crossbites.* Care is needed to avoid arbitrary correction of molar crossbites by tipping movements (**282**).

This allows extrusion of palatal cusps and unwanted opening of the mandibular plane angle in the treatment of high-angle, and even routine, Class II division 1 problems. Whenever possible, molar crossbites should be corrected by bodily movement.

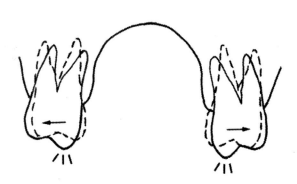

282 Expansion of upper inter-molar width by arbitrary tipping, with consequent extrusion of palatal cusps, represents a lack of vertical molar control. Bodily movement is preferable.

An assessment of maxillary bone can be made, and if it is too narrow, early rapid expansion should be considered as a separate procedure prior to leveling and aligning (see **682–686**). If adequate maxillary bone exists, a fixed quadhe-lix expander can be effectively used. Minimal molar cross-bites can usually be corrected in the final stage of leveling and aligning using rectangular wires which are slightly expanded from the normal form (**283–284**).

283

284

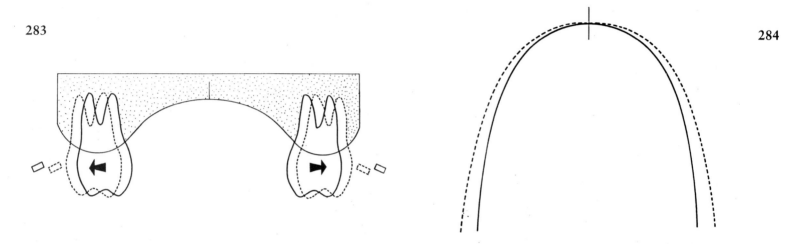

283–284 This figure shows the use of a slightly expanded rectangular wire to achieve correction of a minimal molar crossbite during the final stages of leveling and aligning. Torque control is helpful, to achieve a bodily movement rather than tipping.

Miscellaneous Aspects of Leveling and Aligning

Wire sequence

The opening archwires should apply light and gentle forces, and all wires are bent to archform. The wire sequence used by the authors is as follows: .015 twistflex, .0175 twistflex, .014, .016, .018, .020 round wires, and then .019/.025 rectangular.

The exact sequence varies with the complexity of the mal-occlusion. In difficult cases a particular size may be maintained for more than one month, whereas in easier cases it is often possible to skip a wire size. Nickel titanium wires can be used during various stages of leveling and aligning. However, their two primary disadvantages are their cost, and their flexibility, which can lead to their being inappropriately extended during leveling and aligning (see **277**).

Excessively deflecting these wires to include teeth well out of the archform (in the horizontal or vertical plane) causes distortion of the archform and changes in the plane of occlusion as described above. It is also difficult to put accurate bendbacks into nickel titanium wires.

Exceptions to Full Bracket Placement

Placement of brackets or bands on all possible teeth is recommended at the start of most treatments. This allows for the earliest possible stabilization of archform and also helps control the cuspids during their initial retraction. The exceptions to full bracket placement are as follows:

- *High angle deep bite cases in which the upper incisors interfere with bracket placement on the lower incisors.*

These cases are unusual, but when they occur, the upper incisors can be bracketed and the lower incisors left unbracketed at the start of treatment. After leveling and aligning has occurred in the upper arch for 2-3 months and the upper incisors have been slightly advanced, the lower incisors can then be bracketed. This prevents unnecessary extrusion of posterior teeth during the leveling procedure. In low angle deep bite cases a biteplate can be considered and lower incisor brackets can be placed at the initial banding visit, provided the occlusion allows this.

- *Cases with unerupted teeth, or teeth significantly out of the archform.*

Such teeth can be left unbracketed until adequate space is provided for their movement. Once space is created, these teeth can be bracketed and lightly tied with elastic thread to the main archwire. Sufficient space must be opened for movement of instanding teeth so that they do not fulcrum at the contact area, causing improper root positioning. The creation of adequate space allows bodily movement of these teeth into the archform and more correct root positioning, reducing the treatment needs in the finishing phase (285).

Previously unerupted second molars can be banded at a later stage of treatment. In extraction cases, for example, it may not be beneficial to return to light archwires to include second molars until after major movements (space closure and overjet reduction), have been completed.

- *When cuspids are upright or distally inclined.*

The tip built into the cuspid brackets creates an incisally inclined slot position as shown in 276. As the archwire passes through these bracket slots, it tends to be deflected incisally to the incisor bracket slots. If this archwire is put into the incisor brackets, it has a tendency to extrude these teeth. This effect is greater in the upper arch due to the increased tip in the upper canine brackets. If this is undesirable, and it usually is, then it is better not to bracket the incisors until the cuspid roots have been distalized, making the cuspid slots more parallel to the occlusal plane (286).

285

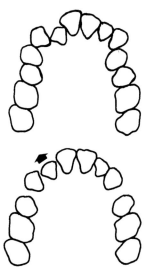

286

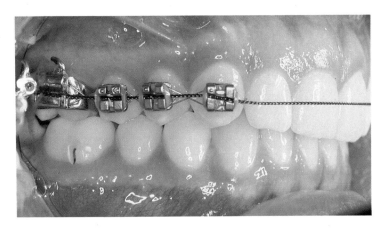

285 Correct technique for alignment of an instanding incisor. If enough space is first created, and a gentle proclining force applied, the tooth will move almost bodily into alignment. If heavy force is applied, before adequate space is provided, the tooth crown will tip labially and the root will move palatally.

286 When cuspids are upright or distally inclined, it may be better not to bracket the incisors at the start of treatment.

Re-leveling Procedures

It is necessary to repeat leveling and aligning procedures in most cases when using preadjusted appliances. Re-leveling is needed when newly erupted teeth are included for the first time, or when bracket or bands are re-cemented, either due to breakage or incorrect original positioning. During treatment, re-leveling should be carried out as few times as possible for treatment efficiency, but even experienced clinicians fail to place all brackets accurately at their first attempt. During early leveling and aligning, these errors can be identified, and it is better to reposition brackets rather than making archwire bends throughout subsequent treatment. Two techniques were found helpful in dealing with brackets which required repositioning:

- Introducing archwire bends at the .014 round wire stage, to compensate for the error (287). This wire shows enough flexibility to produce minor changes in tooth position and the brackets can be repositioned at the next visit. Often .016 round wires can then be placed, without wasting any treatment time. If bracket re-positioning is delayed until the finishing and detailing stage of treatment, then it is necessary to drop from the rectangular wires back to very light wires. This increases the treatment time.

- Repositioning of improperly positioned brackets can also be done when newly erupted or poorly positioned teeth are bracketed, because it is necessary to return to lighter archwires to pick up these teeth. Also, if second molars have not been banded until after a later stage of treatment, such as space closure, or overjet reduction, brackets can be repositioned at the second molar banding visit and the re-leveling procedure can occur without loss of treatment time.

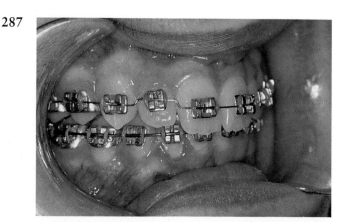

287

287 In this case the upper right lateral incisor bracket was positioned too gingivally during the initial set-up. A compensating step was placed in the .014 archwire. When the bracket was repositioned correctly, it was possible to move forwards into a .016 round wire, with no loss of treatment time.

Key Points during Leveling and Aligning

- Sagittal, vertical, and lateral anchorage needs should be identified for each case.
- Lacebacks should be used to control canine crowns where necessary.
- Bendbacks should be used to prevent proclination of incisors where necessary.
- Posterior segments should be supported with headgear, and/or soldered palatal or lingual bars, in maximal anchorage cases.
- Forces should be light (150 Gm or less).
- The .014 wires (or smaller) should be used until all brackets are correctly placed, before moving into larger sizes.
- Leveling and aligning is not complete until the .019/.025 rectangular steel wire is passive in the brackets. Sliding mechanics should not be attempted before this.

CASE REPORT MM

A Class I four premolar extraction case,
with moderate crowding and
significant protrusion

This 21 year old female presented with a Class I skeletal and dental pattern. She showed an average lower facial height, with significant protrusion of upper and lower incisors, and moderate crowding.

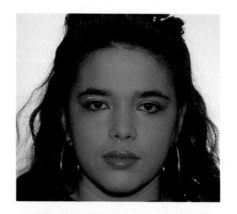

288

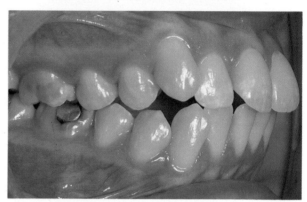

291

Occlusal views confirm that there was substantial crowding of incisors. The teeth were rather wedge-shaped.

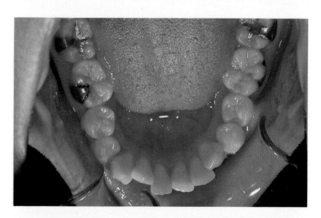

294

Four first premolars were extracted, and anchorage control was used to help achieve a satisfactory result. A headgear was fitted, but co-operation was not good in the first six to nine months.It was decided to band canines, with lingual cleats, to assist rotation control.

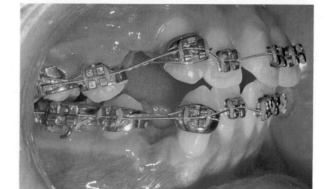

297

289

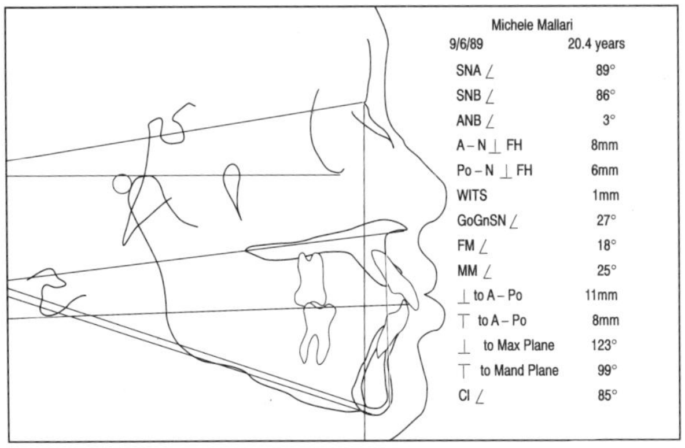

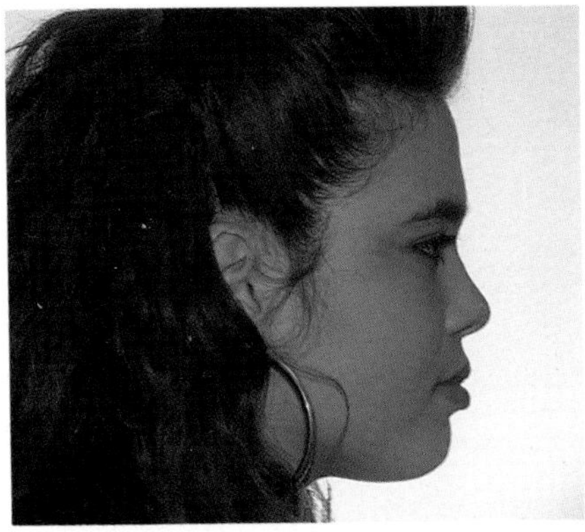

290

Michele Mallari	
9/6/89	20.4 years
SNA ∠	89°
SNB ∠	86°
ANB ∠	3°
A – N ⊥ FH	8mm
Po – N ⊥ FH	6mm
WITS	1mm
GoGnSN ∠	27°
FM ∠	18°
MM ∠	25°
⊥ to A – Po	11mm
⊤ to A – Po	8mm
⊥ to Max Plane	123°
⊤ to Mand Plane	99°
CI ∠	85°

292

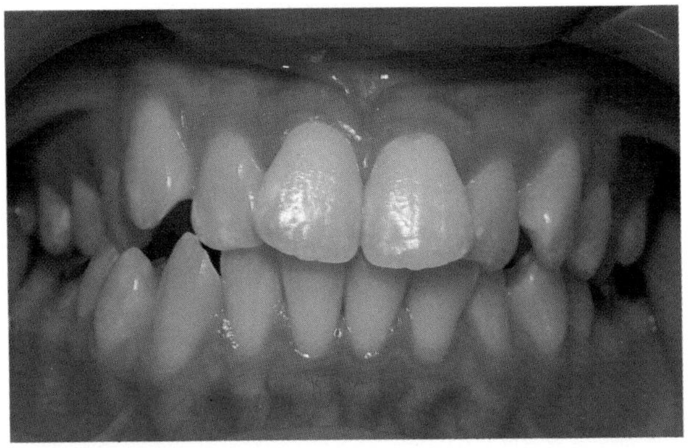

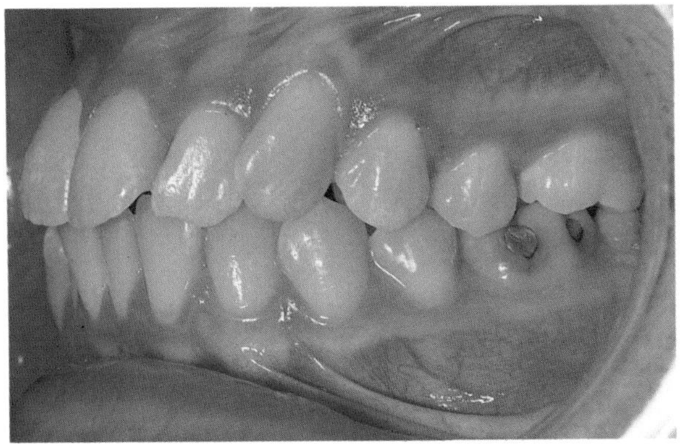

293

295

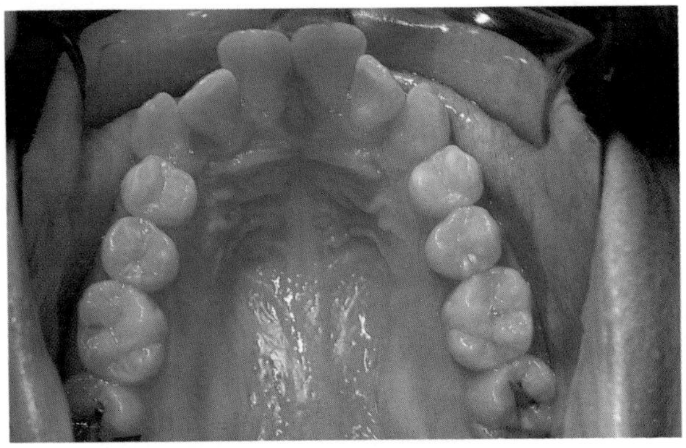

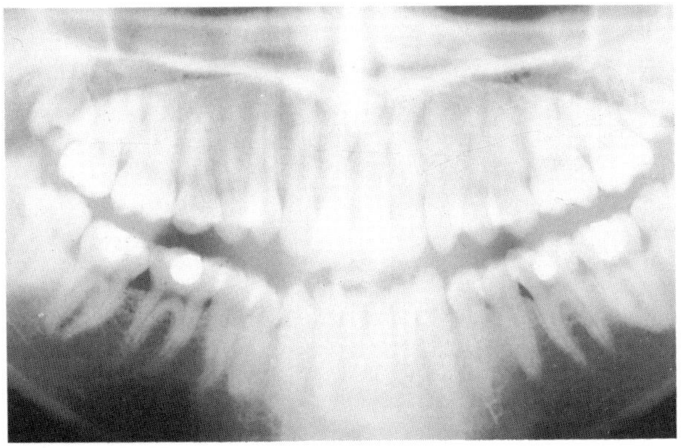

296

298

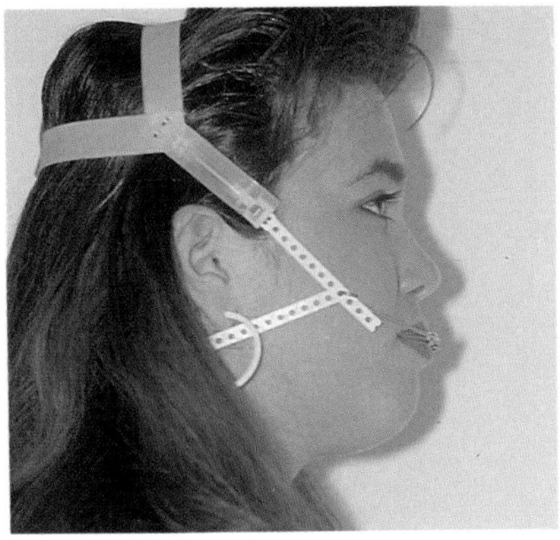

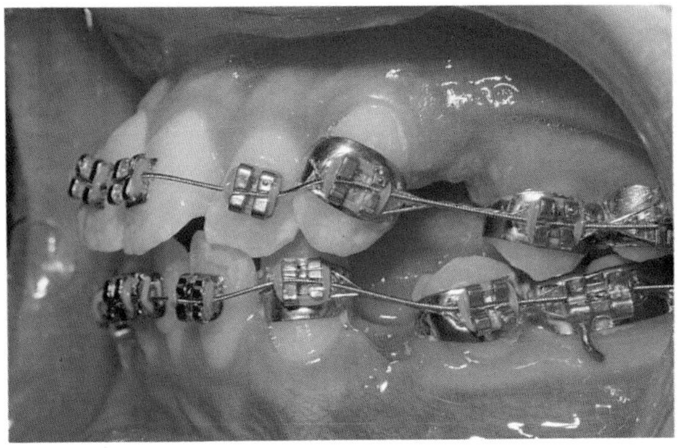

299

A lingual arch and palatal bars were not used, but in retrospect they would have been helpful, due to the initial poor co-operation with headgear.

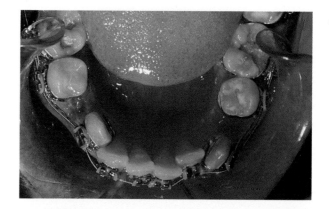

300

Two months into treatment. Lacebacks and bendbacks are being used, with .014 round archwires.

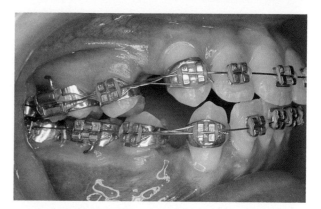

302

After three months of treatment a lower .018 round wire is placed, with passive tiebacks. An upper .020 round wire is in use, with lacebacks and bendbacks.

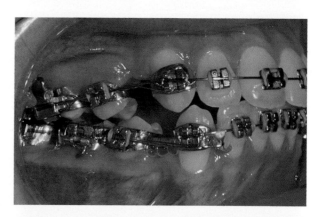

305

Upper and lower archwires are to standard archform.

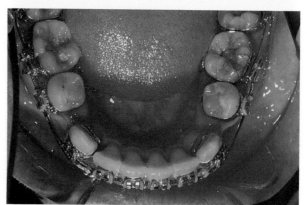

308

301

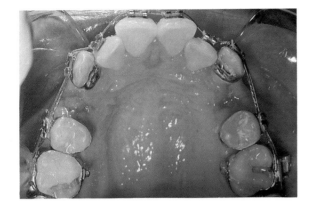

303

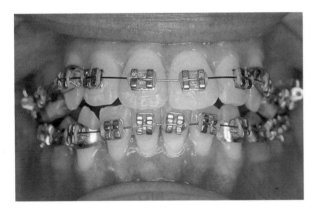

304

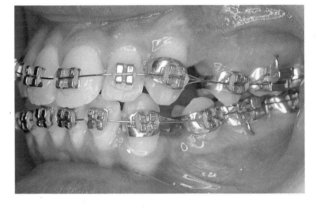

306

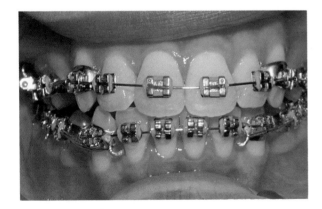

307

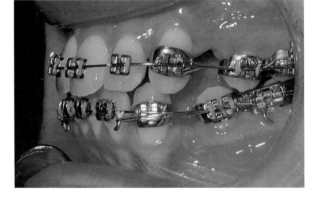

309

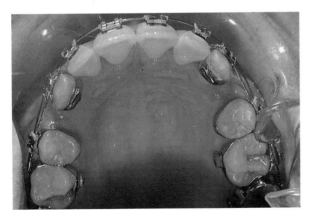

Progress photos and lateral skull X-ray after nine months of treatment. Co-operation with headgear had not been good.

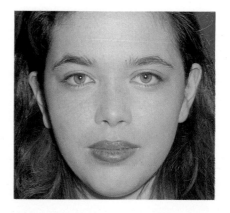

310

Upper arch and lower rectangular .019/.025 wires in place with passive ties. Class III elastics were worn with the headgear, and co-operation improved.

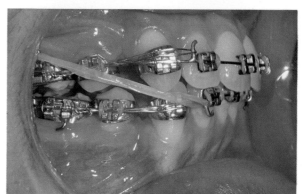

313

After ten months of treatment. Much of the space has closed without the need for active tiebacks, due to lacebacks and passive tiebacks.

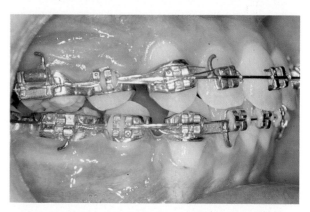

316

Archform has expressed itself.

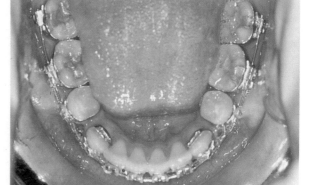

319

311

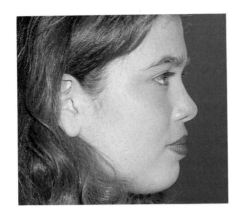

312

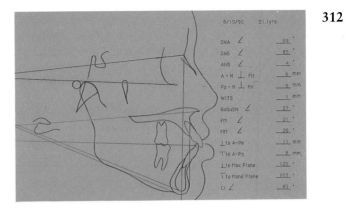

314

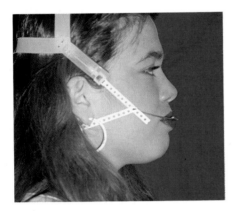

315

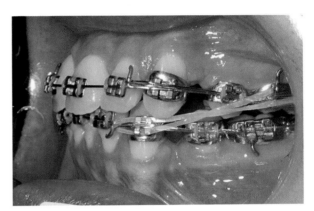

317

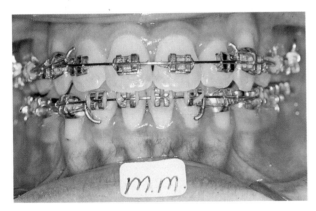

318

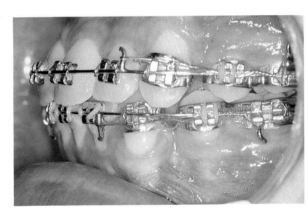

320

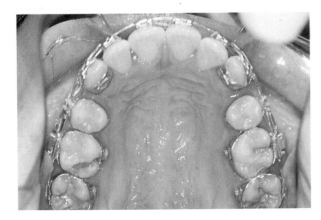

Because of the prominence of upper and lower canines, brackets were placed upside down for these teeth. This created negative torque, to move the roots away from the cortical plate. The authors often use zero torque brackets for canines, as described in Chapter 4 (see **129–130**).

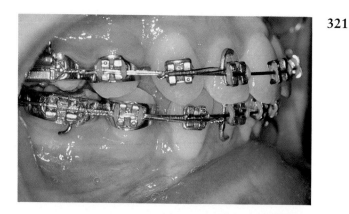

321

Active tiebacks being used to finally close extraction space. In treatment of this young adult at this stage two modules were used with each active tieback, but normally just one module is used.

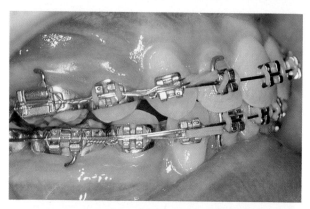

324

Prior to band and bracket removal after 17 months of active treatment.

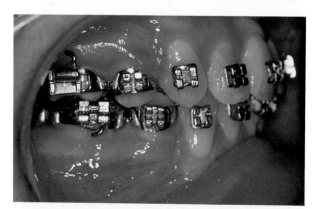

327

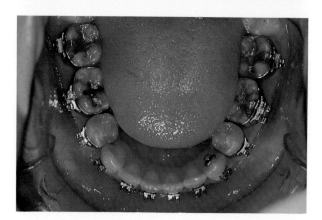

330

322
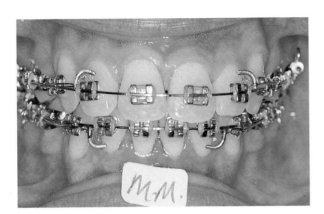

323
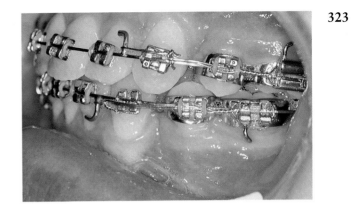

325
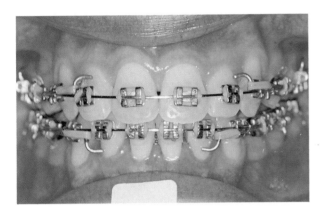

326
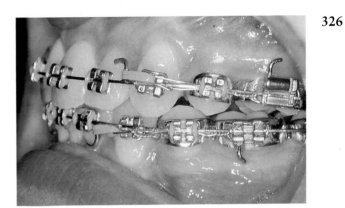

328
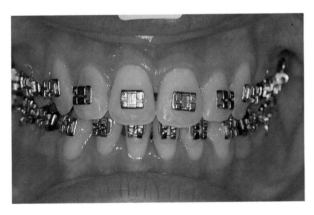

329
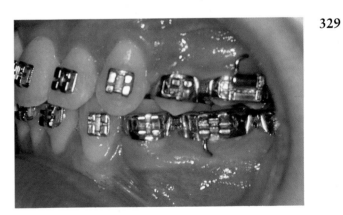

331
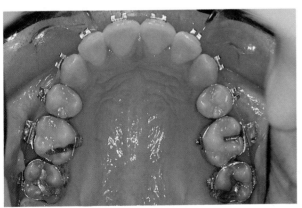

Two months after removal of fixed appliances. The patient wore a nocturnal Hawley retainer in the upper arch and a fixed lower retainer.

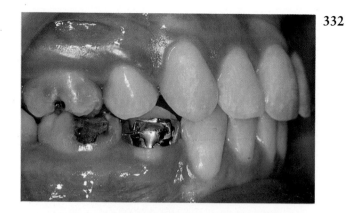

332

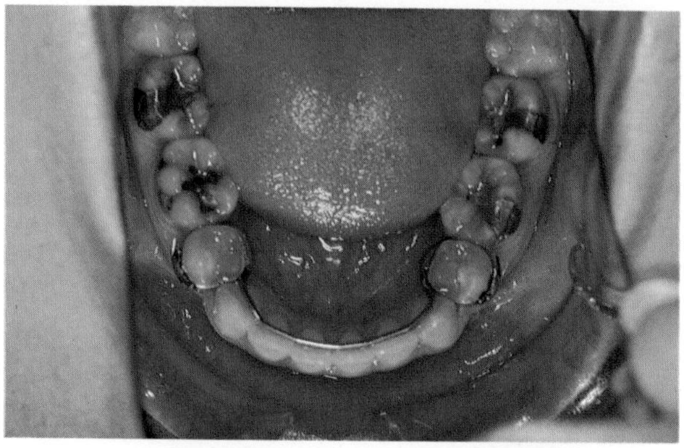

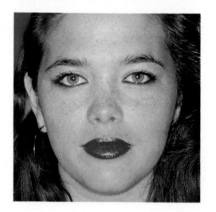

335

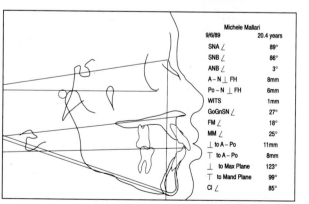

337

Before and after cephalometric tracings; **340** shows superimposition of SN at S.

339

Michele Mallari	
9/6/89	20.4 years
SNA ∠	89°
SNB ∠	86°
ANB ∠	3°
A–N ⊥ FH	8mm
Po–N ⊥ FH	6mm
WITS	1mm
GoGnSN ∠	27°
FM ∠	18°
MM ∠	25°
⊥ to A–Po	11mm
⊤ to A–Po	8mm
⊥ to Max Plane	123°
⊤ to Mand Plane	99°
CI ∠	85°

333

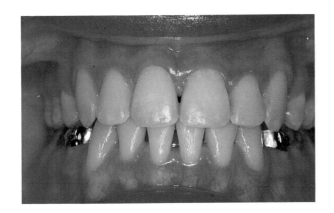

334

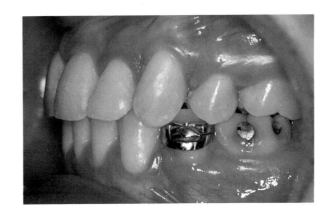

336

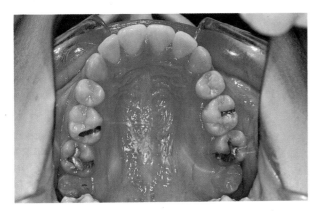

338

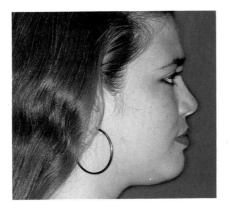

340

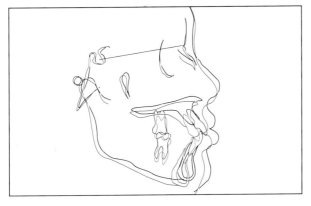

341

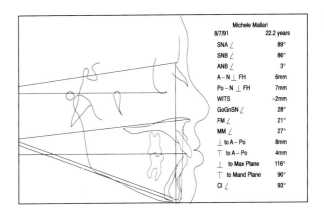

Michele Mallari	
8/7/91	22.2 years
SNA ∠	89°
SNB ∠	86°
ANB ∠	3°
A – N ⊥ FH	6mm
Po – N ⊥ FH	7mm
WITS	–2mm
GoGnSN ∠	28°
FM ∠	21°
MM ∠	27°
⊥ to A – Po	8mm
⊤ to A – Po	4mm
⊥ to Max Plane	116°
⊤ to Mand Plane	90°
CI ∠	93°

The Extraction Decision

The correction of a deep overbite is accomplished by various tooth movements which include the following:

- Extrusion of posterior teeth (342)
- Uprighting of posterior teeth (343)
- Increasing the inclination of incisors (344)
- Intrusion of anterior teeth (345)
- A combination of two or more of the above tooth movements

The main factors to be evaluated for the treatment plan are:

- The vertical dental and skeletal pattern
- The horizontal dental and skeletal pattern
- Protrusion or retrusion of incisors for facial profile reasons
- Upper and lower arch crowding, including curve of Spee, (Steiner's recommendations[3])

The type of tooth movements selected to correct deep overbite depends upon the diagnostic needs of each individual case, and the decision to extract or not extract teeth becomes part of the treatment planning process.

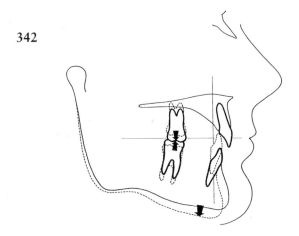

342 Extrusion of posterior teeth.

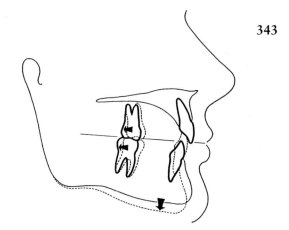

343 Uprighting of posterior teeth.

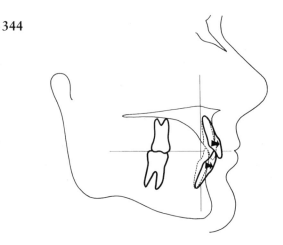

344 Increasing the inclination of incisors.

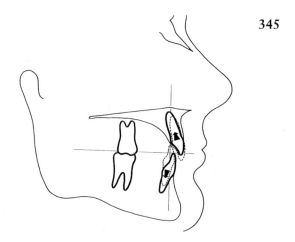

345 Intrusion of anterior teeth.

Vertical Skeletal and Dental Pattern

Proper evaluation of the patient's vertical skeletal and dental pattern is essential in establishing the correct treatment plan for deep overbite cases, and the authors have used the maxillary (palatal) plane to mandibular plane (MM) angle as a key diagnostic measurement. An average of 28° at 12 years of age is used for the MM angle (346).

This measurement is supplemented with the FM angle (average 26°) and the GoGn to SN angle (average 32°).[4] It has been observed that the control of deep overbite in low angle cases (MM angles less than 25°) is easier when non-extraction treatment is carried out. The leveling of the arches and subsequent bite opening with a complete arch system (in such low angle non-extraction cases) occurs primarily as a result of the uprighting and slight extrusion of posterior teeth. The anterior teeth are normally in an upright or retroclined position in these cases. When incisors are slightly advanced or inclined forward, this also encourages bite opening and frequently improves facial esthetics.

The intrusion of anterior teeth is normally not necessary in deep bite cases, since an attempt is usually being made to increase lower facial height rather than to maintain it. The exception to this is the case with retroclined and extruded lower incisors, where an intrusion arch can be used to intrude the incisors prior to their advancement.

If teeth are extracted in low angle deep bite cases, control of the overbite is most difficult. Strong muscle forces make it more difficult for posterior teeth to move anteriorly into extraction sites. As spaces are closed, the anterior teeth then tend to upright as they move posteriorly with subsequent further bite deepening, and undesirable facial profile changes. Thus, unless crowding and/or protrusion is severe in these cases, extraction of teeth is normally avoided. In the very few instances where the extraction of teeth is indicated, leveling and aligning, as well as space closure procedures must be done slowly, with light forces, in order to control the overbite.

High angle deep bite cases (MM angle greater than 31°) present a different set of challenges, with the decision to extract or not extract being more difficult. An attempt should be made to avoid the extrusion of posterior teeth in these unusual cases, in order to avoid further increase in the MM angle and downward and backward rotation of the mandible. This is best accomplished with the use of light forces, supplemented at times with anterior intrusion mechanics. Evaluation of the factors of incisor position and arch crowding become most critical in these cases and there is a greater willingness to consider tooth extraction.

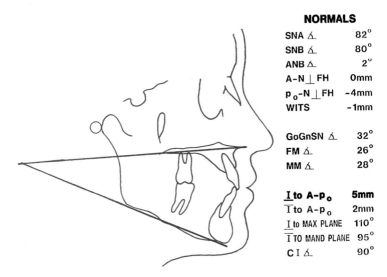

NORMALS

SNA ∡	82°
SNB ∡	80°
ANB ∡	2°
A-N ⊥ FH	0mm
P_o-N ⊥ FH	-4mm
WITS	-1mm
GoGnSN ∡	32°
FM ∡	26°
MM ∡	28°
$\underline{I}$ to A-P_o	5mm
$\overline{I}$ to A-P_o	2mm
$\underline{I}$ to MAX PLANE	110°
$\overline{I}$ TO MAND PLANE	95°
C I ∡	90°

346 Maxillary (palatal) plane to mandibular plane angle (MM) is a key diagnostic measurement in deep bite cases.

121

Horizontal Skeletal and Dental Pattern

The correction of deep overbite must also be assessed in the light of the horizontal skeletal and dental pattern of the patient. A discussion of the Class II deep bite case is pertinent here, since it is most frequently the forward positioning of the maxillary dentition relative to the mandibular dentition that allows for the extrusion of anterior teeth and the subsequent development of the deep overbite.

In treating such cases, if lower incisors can be slightly advanced, it minimizes the need for over-retraction of upper incisors (with negative profile changes) and it also initiates the bite opening process. Non-extraction treatment helps this type of lower incisor movement. If teeth are extracted, there is more of a tendency to maintain or upright incisors,

which works against bite opening. In the maxillary arch, the more that upper incisors need to be retracted (creating the tendency for uprighting), the more difficult it is to correct the deep overbite. The advantage of treating the growing patient versus the non-growing patient, as well as treating on a non-extraction basis, becomes obvious.

When upper teeth need to be extracted in Class II deep bite cases (as with non-cooperating or non-growing patients), great care must be taken to maintain upper incisor torque as these teeth are retracted, and intrusion mechanics to the incisors is sometimes needed to properly allow for bite opening. With severe cases, surgical correction may be the only satisfactory treatment option.

Incisor Position

The evaluation of incisor position using APo line (347) is critical in the management of deep bite cases, as discussed above. When incisors are retrusive and can be advanced, this helps the bite opening process. When they are protrusive and need to be retracted, the bite tends to deepen and the mechanics become more difficult.

Crowding

While evaluation of crowding is important in the treatment planning of deep bite cases, *unless it is severe it does not take precedence over the three factors of vertical dimension, horizontal considerations, and incisor position.* If these three factors favor non-extraction treatment, then all but severely crowded cases can be treated without extractions, using space gaining procedures. These include the uprighting and retraction of molars, the expansion and uprighting of buccal segments, the advancement of incisors, and judicious interproximal stripping. If, on the other hand, the above three factors favor extraction treatment, then even minimally crowded cases can be successfully managed on an extraction basis.

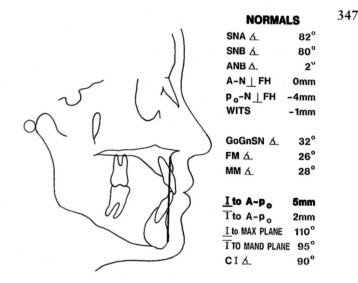

NORMALS		347
SNA ∠	82°	
SNB ∠	80°	
ANB ∠	2°	
A–N ⊥ FH	0mm	
P$_o$–N ⊥ FH	–4mm	
WITS	–1mm	
GoGnSN ∠	32°	
FM ∠	26°	
MM ∠	28°	
I̲ to A–p$_o$	5mm	
I̅ to A–p$_o$	2mm	
I̲ to MAX PLANE	110°	
I̅ TO MAND PLANE	95°	
C I ∠	90°	

347 APo line is used to assess the antero-posterior position of incisors.

Non-extraction Treatment

Most treatment procedures in the management of deep overbite non-extraction cases encourage bite opening. During leveling and aligning with a complete arch system, for example, as progressively larger archwires are placed, the posterior segments are uprighted and slightly extruded while the anterior segments are inclined forward. All of these tooth movements lead to rapid and effective bite opening (see 342, 344, 349).

The use of an upper anterior bite plate is most effective in the initial treatment stages of average to low angle deep bite cases. This appliance relieves posterior muscular forces and encourages the uprighting and extrusion of posterior teeth (348). An anterior bite plate also allows for early placement of brackets on lower incisors, which might otherwise be impossible due to the interference created by the overlap of the upper incisors.

In the treatment of the unusual high angle deep bite cases, the bite plate is contra-indicated since the extrusion of posterior teeth is not desirable. In this situation, brackets can be left off the lower anterior segment until space is available for their placement without interference. Also, in average to low angle deep bite cases, the earliest possible banding of the second molars (especially the lower second molars) is most beneficial in bite opening. It has been observed by the authors in numerous cases that complete leveling of the curve of Spee in the lower arch is virtually impossible without the inclusion of the lower second molars (349).

348

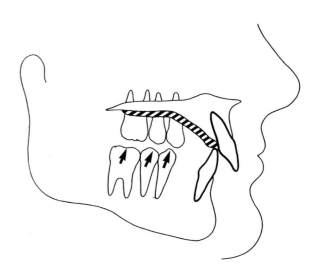

348 The use of an upper anterior bite plate is most effective in the initial leveling stages of average to low angle deep bite cases.

349

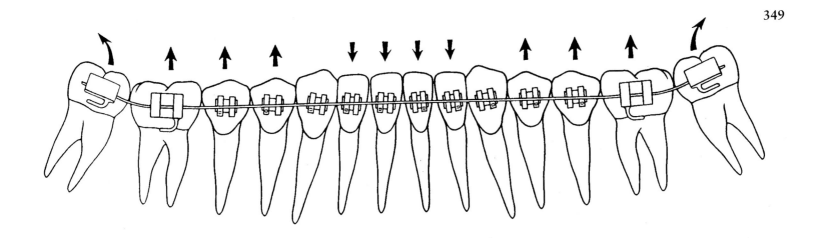

349 In average to low angle deep bite cases, the earliest possible banding of the second molars, especially the lower second molars, is most beneficial in bite opening.

In high angle deep bite cases, it may be decided not to band the upper second molars, to avoid extrusion of these teeth. If they need to be banded for improved positioning or torque control, then the archwire can be stepped up behind the upper first molar to the level of the second molar bracket slot to avoid extrusion.

The leveling and aligning process is often thought of as essentially a round wire procedure that is completed in the very early months of treatment, but it is actually not completed until rectangular wires have been in place for one to three months. It is sometimes even necessary to place minimal bite opening curves in the upper and lower rectangular archwires to complete this stage (350).

The use of a .019/.025 archwire in the .022 bracket slot was found by the authors to be more effective in arch leveling and bite opening than the .017/.025 archwire in the .018 bracket slot.

With the preadjusted appliance system, anchorage control is frequently a concern in the early stages of treatment, since the tip built into the anterior brackets causes these teeth to incline anteriorly. While this movement aids in bite opening, it may or may not be desirable for other reasons, and the use of headgear and light Class III elastics can be helpful in controlling this anterior tipping, as shown in the last chapter.

Class III elastic forces should be very light if used with light leveling wires, to avoid extrusion of the lower incisors and further bite deepening. For this reason, the authors normally wait until they are using at least a .016 round wire to initiate Class III elastics, with force levels of 100 Gms. If anchorage control is needed in these cases for Class II molar correction, and headgear or Class II mechanics are applied to the upper molars, the distalization of these teeth is usually accompanied by some extrusion, which also aids in bite opening.

When overjet reduction is required in the management of deep overbite non-extraction cases, it is most important that bite opening procedures be completed, or at least be well on their way towards completion, prior to the initiation of this next stage of treatment. The premature use of Class II elastics, before the bite is opened, can lead to bite deepening and to excessively heavy interferences between the advancing lower incisors and the retracting upper incisors.

350

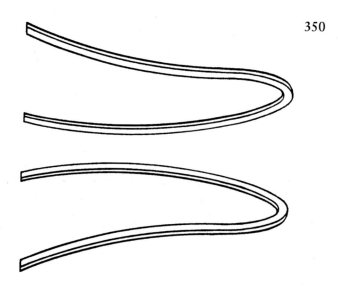

350 Minimal bite opening curves (reverse curve in the lower archwire and accentuated curve in the upper archwire) in rectangular archwires are sometimes beneficial in bite opening, but not necessary in all cases.

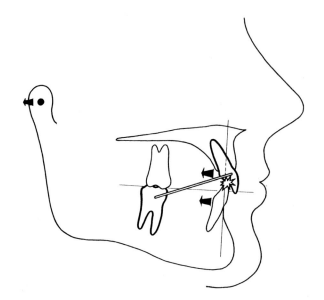

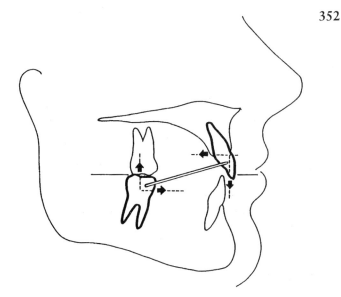

351 Premature attempts at overjet correction, prior to proper overbite control, can lead to excessive and unnecessary anterior contacts, with resultant posterior condylar displacement.

352 Force vectors involved in the use of Class II elastics. The extrusive force on the lower posterior teeth encourages bite opening. Intrusive forces applied to the upper anterior segment (such as accentuated archwire curve or in severe cases 'J' hook headgear) can be used to counteract the extrusive bite deepening effect of Class II elastics on the upper anterior segment.

This in turn can lead to periodontal breakdown, tooth wear, or root resorption of the incisors, as well as a tendency to distally displace the mandible (351).

Orthodontists are being called upon to avoid potentially damaging forces to the temporomandibular joints, and avoidance of premature use of Class II elastics is one significant way of minimizing these forces. This principle is particularly applicable to deep bite extraction cases, where bite opening is more difficult. When bite opening has been adequately controlled, overjet reduction can proceed effectively with the use of headgears and/or Class II elastics. Class II elastics are particularly effective during this stage of treatment in average to low angle cases, because the extrusive force applied to the lower posterior segment encourages the completion and maintenance of bite opening (352).

In high angle deep bite cases, Class II elastics should be used minimally, and with light force, to avoid the extrusion of posterior teeth.

Space Closure

Normally, this is not difficult with the non-extraction deep bite cases. When minimal spacing does occur, it can be easily closed after leveling and bite opening procedures have been completed in these cases.

Extraction Treatment

Most of the treatment procedures described for deep bite non-extraction cases also apply to deep bite extraction cases. These include the effective use of bite plates, second molar banding, the use of the .022 slot versus the .018 slot, the use of headgear and Class III elastics for anchorage control and their effect on overbite control, and the importance of proper overbite control prior to the use of Class II mechanics for overjet reduction. There are two other important factors in extraction deep bite cases:

- With extraction cases, orthodontists are most frequently maintaining or uprighting incisors, which makes bite opening more difficult.
- The tendency to attempt space closure before properly leveling and controlling the overbite, leads to further bite deepening.

One of the great advantages of the preadjusted appliance system is sliding mechanics. This was not possible with the standard edgewise appliance due to the posterior archwire bends, and loops in the archwires.

In order for the rectangular archwire to effectively slide through the posterior bracket slots of a preadjusted appliance, these segments must be free of friction. This need for a *friction free system* relates to all the principles that have been recommended for proper leveling and overbite control, for without these, the archwires cannot slide through the posterior bracket slots. When archwires are in a deflected state, due to incomplete leveling of the arches (incomplete leveling of the curve of Spee), they cannot effectively slide through the posterior bracket slots during space closure, due to the friction in the system. The authors have found that effective correction of deep overbite in extraction cases requires the use of light force levels during leveling and aligning and during space closure.

Light Forces During Leveling and Aligning

When premolars are extracted in deep bite cases, it is normally to reduce anterior protrusion, eliminate anterior crowding, or for a combination of these two reasons. Management of the canines is important.

When anterior protrusion occurs without crowding, it is possible to retract the anterior segments en masse. Alternatively, the canines can be retracted alone, followed by retraction of the incisors.

If the latter decision is made, extreme care must be taken not to tip the the cuspids distally, because this results in extrusion of the incisors and further bite deepening. For this reason, the authors prefer to carry out en masse retraction of the anterior six teeth with a rectangular wire, after arch leveling and overbite control.

Some orthodontists believe that it helps to maintain anchorage if the canines are retracted separately, and then the incisors are retracted, but there seems to be little evidence to support this hypothesis, and most certainly treatment time is increased if this is done. Also, a second major area of gingival tissue and alveolar bone is created with this technique, between the lateral incisors and the canines, and this must be carefully managed.

In cases with anterior crowding, it is necessary to retract the canines until there is enough space for proper incisor alignment. It is then possible, later in the treatment, to carry out en masse movement of the anterior segment. The authors prefer not to retract canines away from the lateral incisors, for the reasons described above.

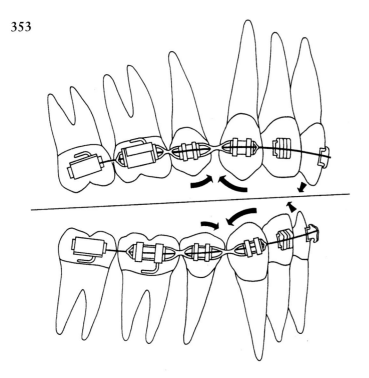

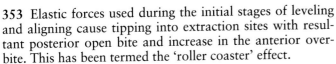

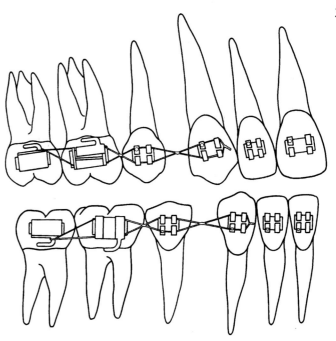

353 Elastic forces used during the initial stages of leveling and aligning cause tipping into extraction sites with resultant posterior open bite and increase in the anterior overbite. This has been termed the 'roller coaster' effect.

354 'Lacebacks' are .009 or .010 figure eight ligature wires extended from molars to canines. They prevent anterior tipping of the canines and can effectively retract them without distal tipping.

There is a tendency for incisors and canines to tip mesially, after placement of the opening archwires. This is caused by the built-in tip features of the preadjusted appliance system. The authors have previously stated that elastic forces should not be used at this early stage, because the canines tend to tip distally and the overbite tends to increase. This is accompanied by posterior bite opening and the overall reaction has been called the 'roller coaster' effect (**353**) which increases the treatment time. For this reason 'lacebacks' have been used to prevent anterior tipping of the canines and to retract these teeth without distal tipping (**354**).

The lacebacks initially compress the periodontal ligament space on the distal aspect of the canine, leading to slight tipping. This is followed by adequate time for uprighting, in response to the leveling effect of the archwire. This uprighting occurs with a laceback, but it is not seen if elastic chains are used, because they give a continuous force which does not allow time for rebound to occur.

355

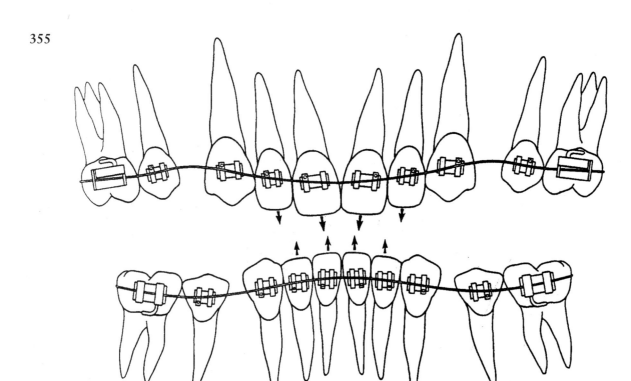

355 If preadjusted brackets are placed on upright or distally tipped canines, an extrusive effect is created on the incisors after the initial archwires have been placed.

The discussion so far has assumed a favorable initial position of the canine teeth, with the crowns at slight or moderate anterior inclination. However, if the canines show unfavorable angulation at the start of treatment, much greater care is needed to ensure good overbite control. Figure 355 shows how preadjusted brackets, on unfavorably angled canines, can cause unwanted extrusion of incisors after the initial archwires have been placed.

The authors normally prefer to bracket as many incisors as possible and to attach them to the initial archwires, to provide greater stability of the archform. However, when canines are unfavorably angled, they sometimes prefer not to involve the incisors until the canine roots have been retracted, providing more favorable angulation of the canine slots. This technique minimizes the inevitable tendency for bite deepening in such cases.

In summary, it is clear that there are many factors which can lead to bite deepening during the initial leveling stage. Effective overbite control requires the use of light forces, with minimal activation and adequate rebound time. Lacebacks have proved to be the most effective way of controlling canine position and movement, and hence the overbite in these cases.

Light Forces During Space Closure

356

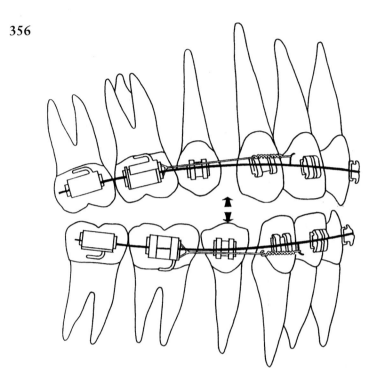

357

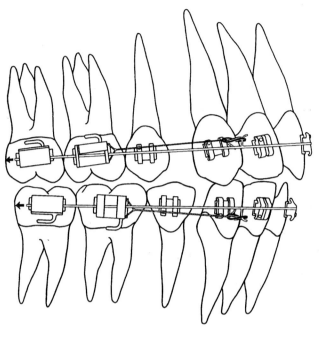

356 Excessive forces applied to rectangular wires during space closure lead to the following negative effects: archwire deflection and binding, ineffective sliding mechanics, loss of anterior torque control and bite deepening.

357 Active tiebacks. Elastic modules attached to anterior archwire hooks, with ligature wires extended from molars, deliver light and effective space closing forces.

In the management of deep bite extraction cases, it has been shown that there is a tendency for the overbite to deepen during the leveling and aligning stage. This same tendency occurs during space closure with rectangular wires, if forces are excessive. Such heavy forces cause the bite to deepen in two ways:

- The canines tip into the extraction sites causing archwire deflection and binding; the sliding mechanics then become ineffective and the overbite deepens.
- Excessive forces overpower the torque control of the rectangular wire on the incisors, particularly the uppers (**356**), causing distal tipping and bite deepening.

For this reason, a small amount of torque added to the upper archwire in the incisor region, combined with lighter forces, is usually found to be effective in minimizing these two bite deepening factors.

The authors have tried various force levels during space closure and feel that a range of 50–150 g is most effective. It minimizes the bite deepening effect, and allows for efficient sliding mechanics and space closure. A small elastic module attached to an anterior archwire hook, with a ligature wire extended forward from a molar, was found to be most effective in delivering a force of this size (**357**). This is called an 'active tieback'.

Summary

This chapter explains some of the measures which the authors use when correcting deep overbites with preadjusted appliances. Specifically, it recommends that good control can be obtained in most cases, if the following are observed:

- The avoidance of elective extractions in low angle cases whenever possible.
- The use of .022 slot brackets, with .019/.025 working rectangular wires.
- The use of anterior acrylic bite plates in average to low angle deep bite cases at the beginning of treatment.
- Light forces at the start of treatment, to avoid overbite deepening.
- The avoidance of elastic retraction forces with canine brackets.
- The banding or bracketing of second molars as early as possible.
- The selective use of Class II elastics.
- The unhurried final leveling of upper and lower arches, using flat rectangular wires initially, before introducing bite opening curves if needed.
- Gentle space closure forces in extraction cases.

CASE REPORT CF

A low angle deep overbite case, with a Class I skeletal and dental pattern

This thirteen and a half year old girl presented with a Class I skeletal pattern, and a deep incisor overbite, showing some of the features of Class II division 2 malocclusion, with a typical high lip line. Treatment was on a non-extraction basis, with leveling and aligning of the arches and a short phase of Class II elastics.

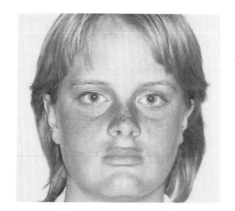

358

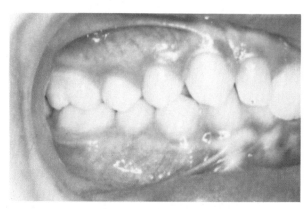

361

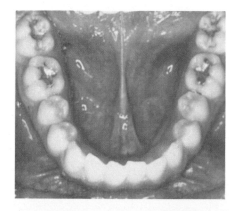

364

An acrylic bite plate was used to help in the early stages of bite opening and leveling and aligning.

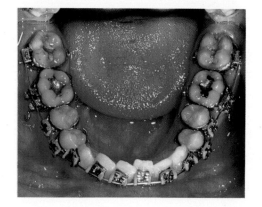

367

359

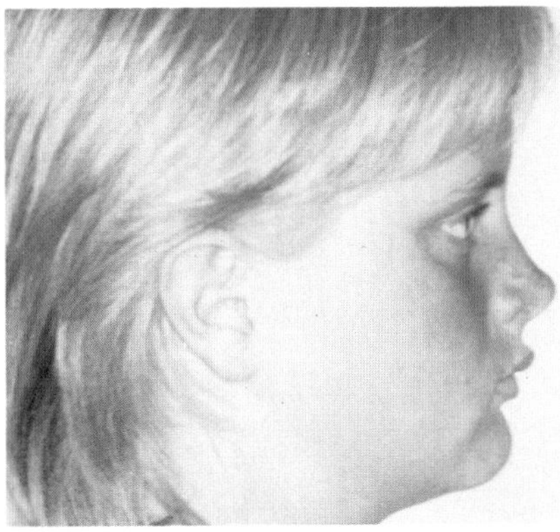

360

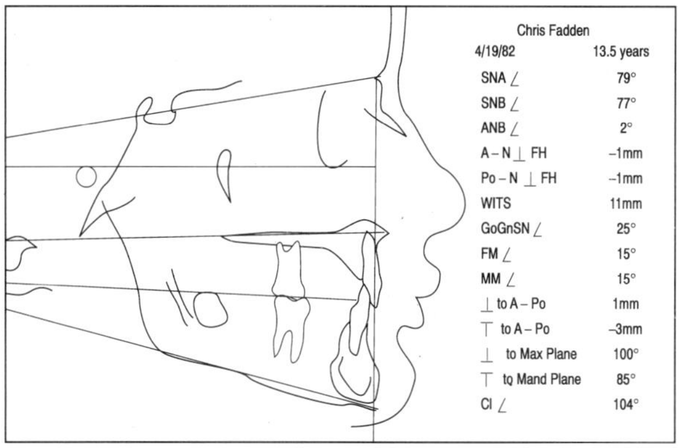

Chris Fadden	
4/19/82	13.5 years
SNA ∠	79°
SNB ∠	77°
ANB ∠	2°
A – N ⊥ FH	–1mm
Po – N ⊥ FH	–1mm
WITS	11mm
GoGnSN ∠	25°
FM ∠	15°
MM ∠	15°
⊥ to A – Po	1mm
⊤ to A – Po	–3mm
⊥ to Max Plane	100°
⊤ to Mand Plane	85°
CI ∠	104°

362

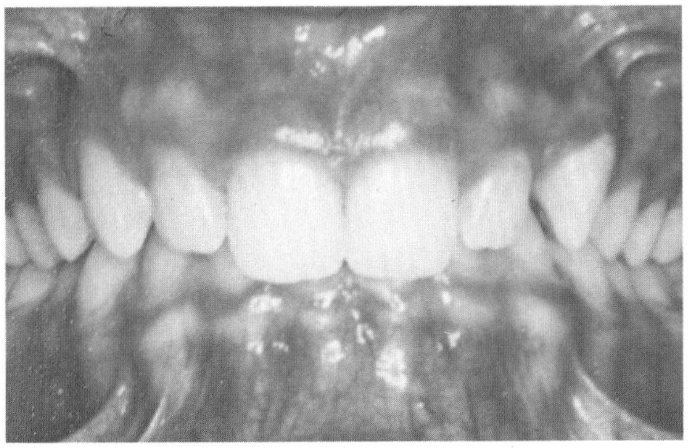

363

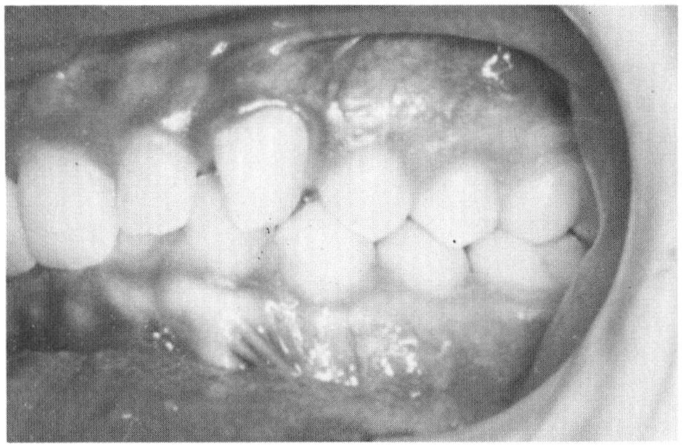

365

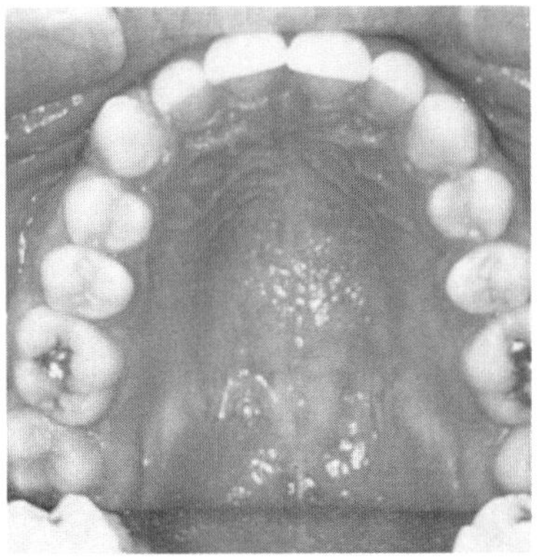

366

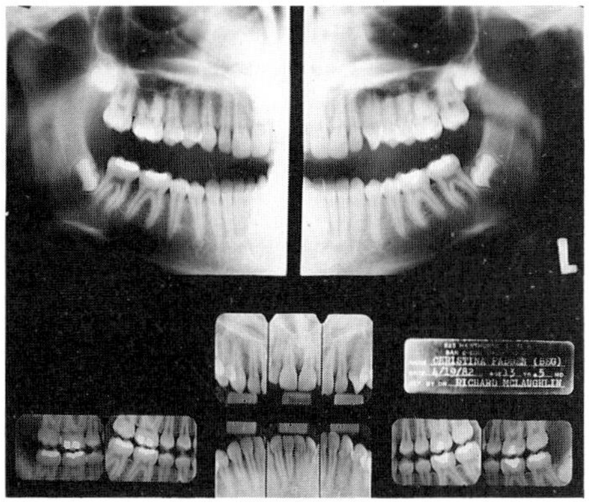

368

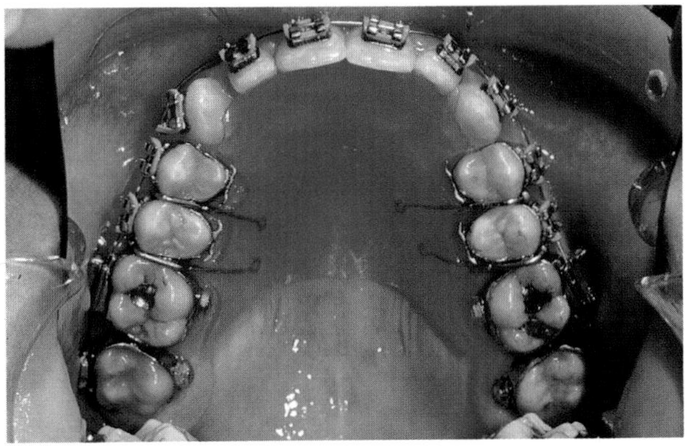

369

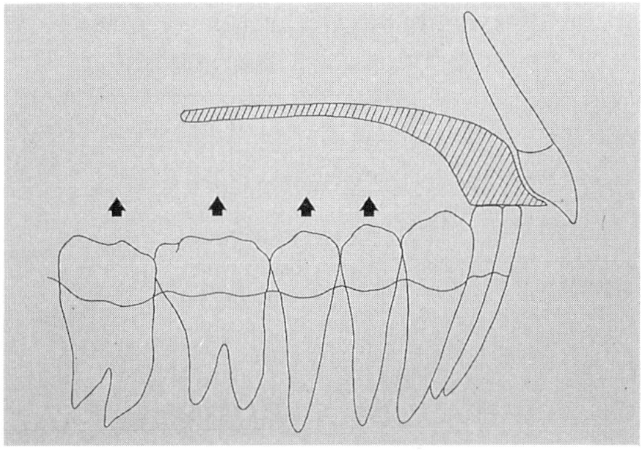

Soon after the start of treatment, with early leveling and aligning archwires.

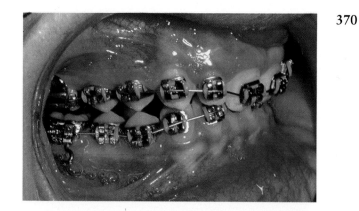

370

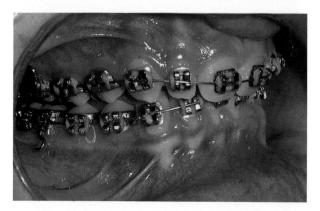

373

After five months of treatment. Upper and lower rectangular archwires are in place, with gently active tiebacks to prevent space opening as incisor torque takes place.

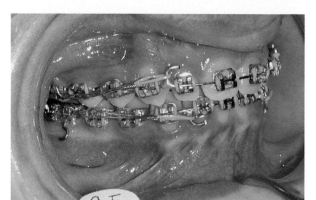

376

Extra torque was added to the upper archwire later in treatment. Full banding, including the second molars, allowed good overbite control.

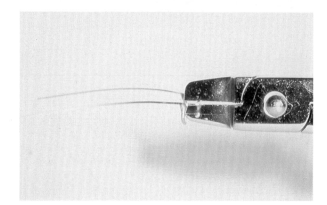

379

371
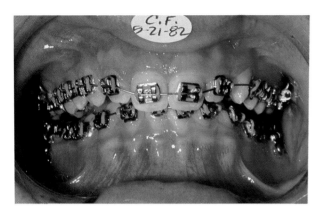

372
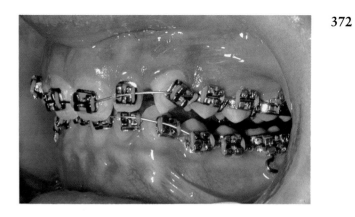

374
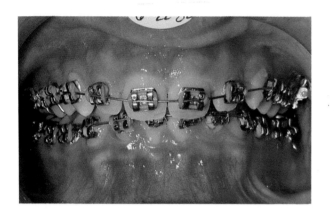

375
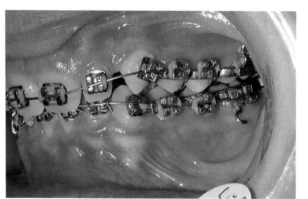

377
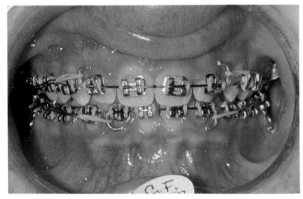

378
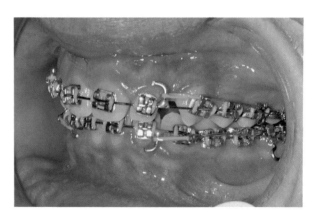

380
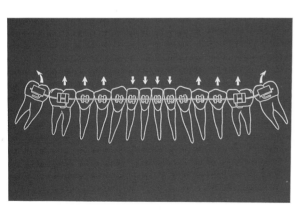

381
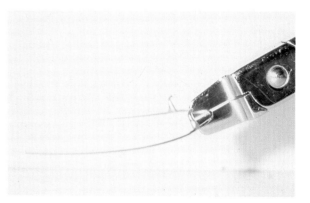

Close to the end of treatment. Upper incisors are tied with wire ligatures for full expression of the bracket features.

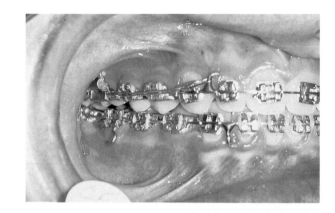

382

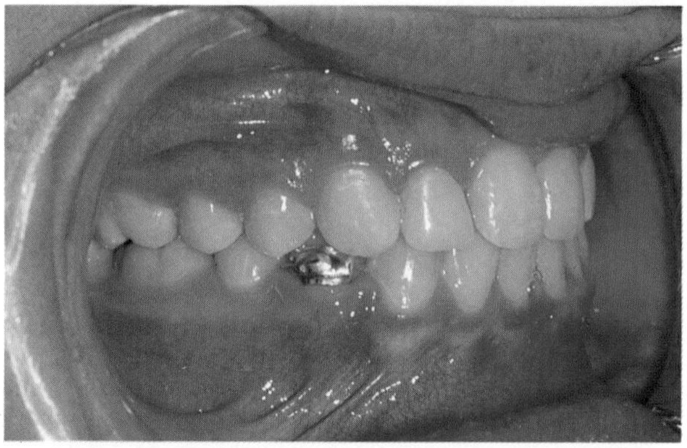

385

A lower premolar-to-premolar retainer was placed. The patient wore an upper Hawley retainer at night.

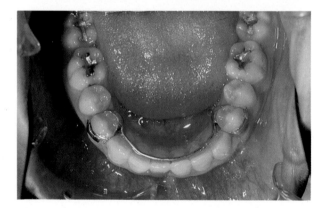

388

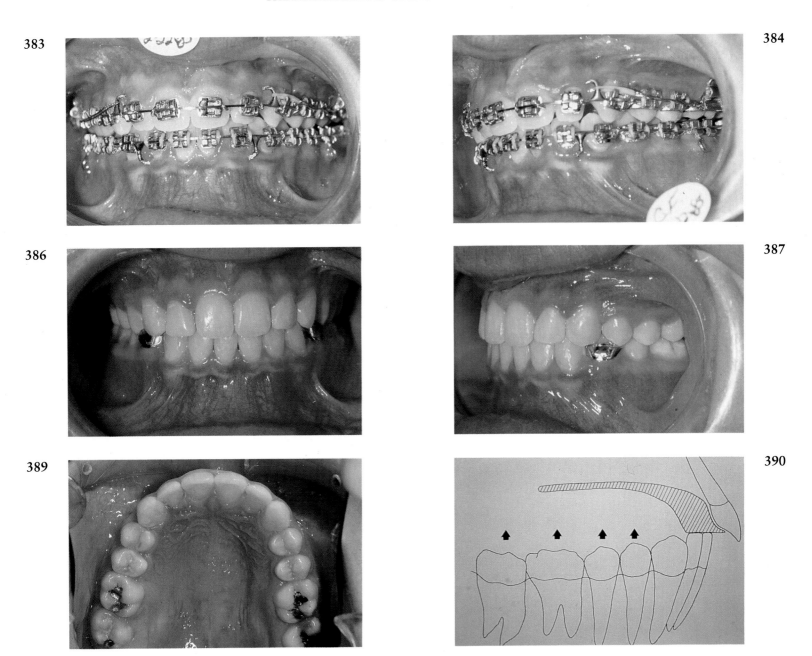

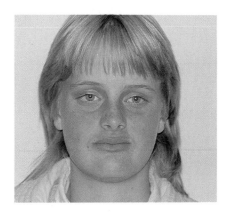

391

Before and after cephalometric tracings show that successful overbite control was achieved by a change in lower incisor angulation from 85° to 97°, and upper incisor angulation from 100° to 120°.

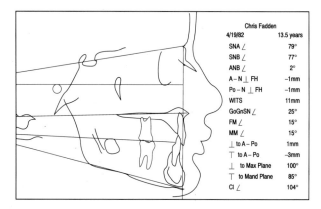

394

Chris Fadden	
4/19/82	13.5 years
SNA ∠	79°
SNB ∠	77°
ANB ∠	2°
A – N ⊥ FH	–1mm
Po – N ⊥ FH	–1mm
WITS	11mm
GoGnSN ∠	25°
FM ∠	15°
MM ∠	15°
⊥ to A – Po	1mm
T to A – Po	–3mm
⊥ to Max Plane	100°
T to Mand Plane	85°
CI ∠	104°

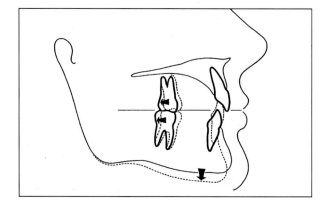

397

392

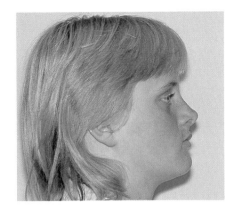

393

STAGES OF TREATMENT

1 **Anchorage control**
2 **Leveling & aligning**
3 **Overbite control**
4 **Overjet reduction**
5 **Space closure**
6 **Finishing and detailing**

395

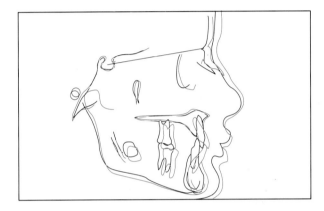

396

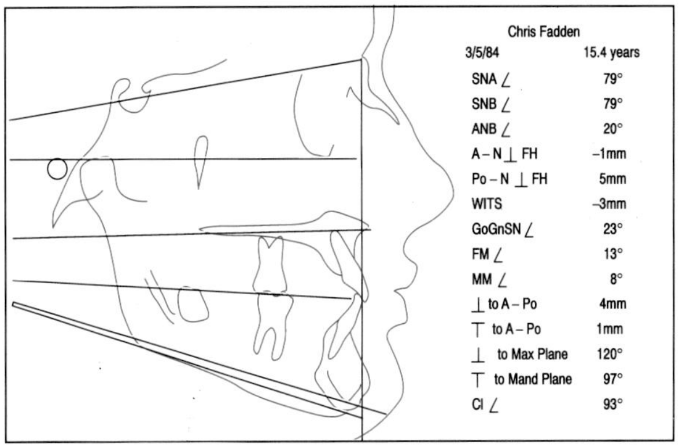

Chris Fadden	
3/5/84	15.4 years
SNA ∠	79°
SNB ∠	79°
ANB ∠	20°
A – N ⊥ FH	–1mm
Po – N ⊥ FH	5mm
WITS	–3mm
GoGnSN ∠	23°
FM ∠	13°
MM ∠	8°
⊥ to A – Po	4mm
⊤ to A – Po	1mm
⊥ to Max Plane	120°
⊤ to Mand Plane	97°
Ci ∠	93°

398

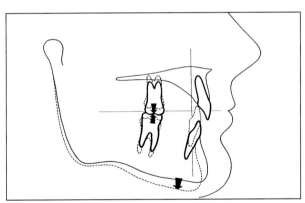

399

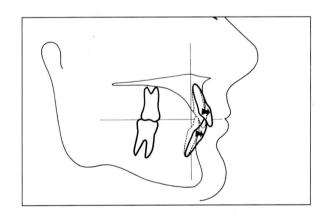

9. OVERJET REDUCTION

Dental and Skeletal Changes Responsible for Overjet Reduction

In previous chapters the various stages of orthodontic treatment have been discussed with special reference to the use of preadjusted appliance systems. One key stage of treatment is overjet reduction, which is required in a large number of cases. The purpose of this chapter is to discuss overjet reduction without surgical intervention, and examples will then be shown of treatment mechanics in typical clinical situations. The following cephalometric measurements (**400**) will be used throughout, and are based on averages from *An Atlas of Craniofacial Growth*,[1] and on the recommendations of Steiner, McNamara, and Jacobson.[2–4] The four non-surgical changes responsible for overjet reduction are:

- Mesial movement of lower incisors.
- Distal movement of upper incisors.
- Distalizing or limiting the forward growth of the maxilla.
- Mesial movement of the mandible due to (a) forward mandibular growth rotation or (b) limiting posterior dental and skeletal vertical development.

Closely tied to overjet reduction is Class II molar correction, which must occur prior to overjet reduction (using headgear to the molars or Class II elastics and sliding jigs to the molars) or at the same time as overjet reduction (as occurs with headgears or Class II elastics to the entire upper arch and with functional appliances). The following four dental and skeletal changes are responsible for Class II molar correction:

- Mesial movement of lower molars.
- Distal movement of upper molars.
- Distalizing or limiting the forward growth of the maxilla.
- Mesial movement of the mandible due to (a) forward mandibular growth rotation or (b) limiting of posterior dental and skeletal vertical development.

Note that first two changes in each of the above lists involve dental tooth movement, while the remaining changes involve skeletal change. In adult non-growing patients, such skeletal changes must be carried out surgically.

400

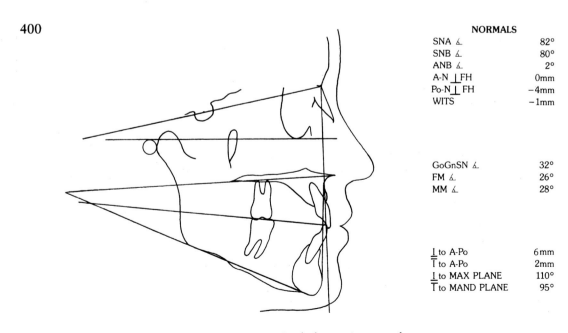

NORMALS	
SNA ∠	82°
SNB ∠	80°
ANB ∠	2°
A-N ⊥FH	0mm
Po-N ⊥ FH	−4mm
WITS	−1mm
GoGnSN ∠	32°
FM ∠	26°
MM ∠	28°
1̲ to A-Po	6mm
1̅ to A-Po	2mm
1̲ to MAX PLANE	110°
1̅ to MAND PLANE	95°

400 Cephalometric normals.

Proper diagnosis of orthodontic cases with Class II molar relationships and/or overjets involves the correct integration of one or more of these dental and skeletal changes.

Each of the changes involved in overjet reduction will be reviewed in detail, and they are shown diagrammatically below (401–5).

401

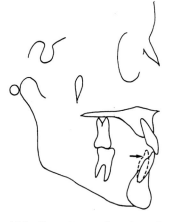

402

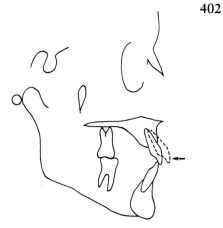

401 Overjet reduction from mesial movement of lower incisors.

402 Overjet reduction from distal movement of upper incisors.

403

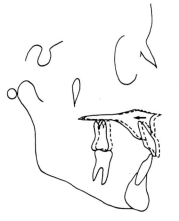

403 Overjet reduction from distalizing or limiting the forward growth of the maxilla.

404

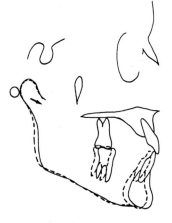

405

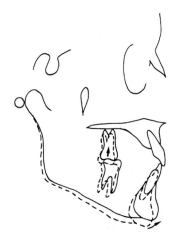

404 Overjet reduction from mesial movement of the body of the mandible resulting from condylar growth.

405 Overjet reduction from mesial movement of the body of the mandible resulting from limiting vertical dental and skeletal development.

Mesial movement of lower incisors

In general, the end-of-treatment position of the lower incisors is important for several reasons. If the lower incisors are too far back, then there is a tendency to a retrognathic profile and a long-term deepening of the overbite (406). If the lower incisors are too far forward, there is undue fullness of the facial profile, together with possible instability of alignment of the lower labial segment, as incisors drop back towards the tongue in response to lip pressure (407).

APo line is useful in the assessment of treatment objectives, using lower incisors at +2 mm as a normal (408), although many other analyses exist and may be preferred by individual orthodontists. The rigid adherence to cephalometric normals relative to lower incisor position is not in the best inter-est of many patients. It must be remembered that this normal is established primarily for the Class I cases and is often modified when dental compensation is needed. For example, in Class III cases the lower incisors may need to be more upright to properly accommodate the upper incisors, and in some Class II cases the lower incisors are best left slightly more forward so that the maxillary incisors do not need to be over-retracted.

It is also conventional to seek a treatment result where the lower incisors are from 90–95° to the mandibular plane, but the ideal for this angle will decrease as MM or FM angles increase and will also vary as dental compensation is required.

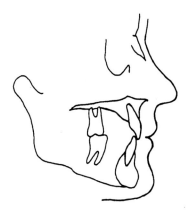

406 The end-of-treatment position of the lower incisors is important for several reasons. If the lower incisors are left too far back, there is a tendency towards a retrognathic profile and a long-term deepening of the overbite.

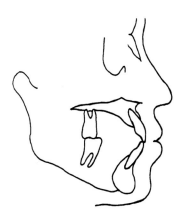

407 If the lower incisors are left too forward, there will be a tendency to undue fullness of the facial profile, together with possible instability of alignment of the lower labial segment.

408

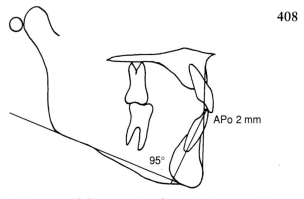

408 APo line is useful in assessing lower incisor position.

There is usually soft tissue involvement in the aetiology of cases which require mesial movement of lower incisors. For example, there may be a history of thumb-sucking activity or hyperactive mentalis muscle function where lower incisors have been held back and retroclined. In these cases, it is mechanically appropriate to move the lower incisors forward (**409**).

Class II, division 2 treatment sometimes involves the mesial movement of lower incisors. There is often a soft tis-
sue element to such cases, where the high lip line with resultant lip activity has retroclined both upper and lower incisors, when compared to normal. During routine mechanics after the upper incisors have been moved forward to create a Class II, division 1 pattern with an overjet, it is frequently found that the lower incisors are back in the profile. It is then appropriate to tip the lower incisors forward to assume a good antero-posterior position in the profile and a favorable interincisal angle (**410, 411**).

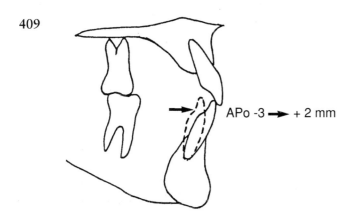

409 APo -3 ➝ + 2 mm

409 Mesial movement of lower incisors after previous thumb sucking activity.

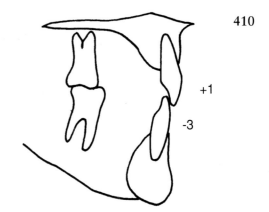

410 +1 -3

410 Class II division 2 incisor relationship at the start of treatment.

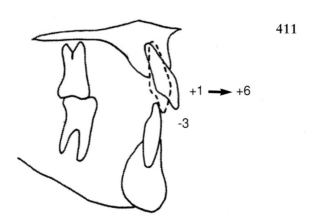

411 +1 ➝ +6 -3

411 Same case as 410, after upper incisor proclination. Adequate upper incisor torque is often a factor in stability. This case will require the lower incisor tooth movement shown in 409 to achieve normal incisor relationship.

Distal movement of upper incisors

The ideal position of the upper incisors may be considered as APo + 6 mm (412) with an angulation of 110° to the maxillary plane, but other evaluation methods and normals exist, which may be preferred by individual orthodontists. If the MM (maxillary or palatal plane to mandibular plane) angle is high, then angulation of the upper incisors to maxillary plane, and lower incisors to mandibular plane, may need to be lower than average, with an increased inter-incisal angle (413).

Traditionally, distal movement of upper incisors has been regarded as the main method of correction of Class II division 1 malocclusions (414). However, since it has been shown that true maxillary protrusion occurs in only about 20% of Class II cases,[5] changes involving mesial movement of chin point are preferable for facial profile reasons. In adults, this implies orthognathic surgery to the maxilla and/or the mandible.

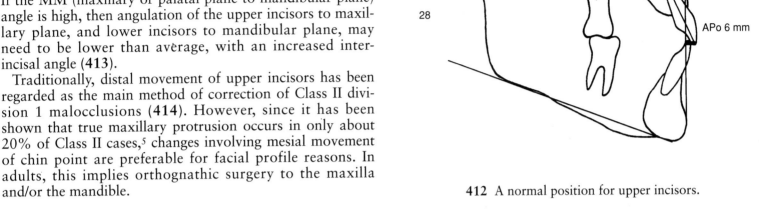

412

412 A normal position for upper incisors.

413

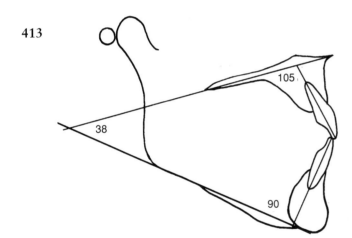

413 Ideals vary as MM angle increases or decreases. If MM is above average, upper and lower incisor angulation will tend to reduce relative to maxillary and mandibular planes, with increased inter-incisal angle. The same dental compensation factors must be considered for the upper incisors as for the lower incisors (more upright in Class II cases and inclined more forward in Class III cases).

414

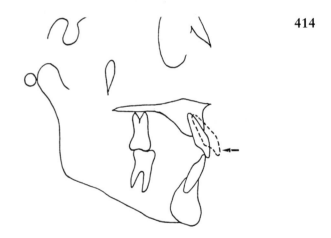

414 Traditionally, distal movement of upper incisors has been the main method of correction of Class II division 1 malocclusion. However, only about 20% of Class II cases have true maxillary protrusion. Therefore, changes involving mesial movement of pogonion point, are usually preferable to optimize facial profile changes.

Where the commencing upper incisor angulation is above 115°, the initial retraction is often achieved by a tipping type of movement until normal angulation is reached, and thereafter bodily movement is attempted. In theory, therefore, round wire may be used during the early stages of this movement. However, rectangular wire is recommended, because if torque is 'lost' and incisor angulation is not controlled, clinical experience has shown that it is difficult to retrieve lost torque. It is better to seek bodily retraction, with good torque control and light forces in cases with a large commencing overjet (**415, 416**).

Also, incisor brackets having additional torque, as suggested in Chapter 3, are recommended in such cases. Archform is a factor. Many Class II division 1 cases have a narrowing of the upper archform before treatment and as this becomes normal during leveling and aligning, there follows a consequential reduction in overjet, provided molar control is maintained (**417, 418**).

415

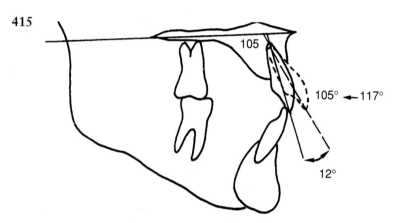

416

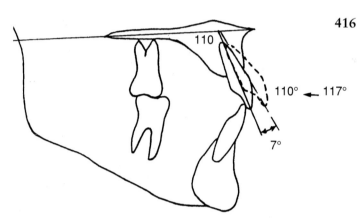

415 Overjet has been reduced, but torque control was not maintained. This will occur if round wire is used for retraction, if retraction is too rapid, or if brackets are placed too incisally. It is mechanically difficult to retrieve this 'lost' torque.

416 Overjet reduction with proper torque control. This requires rectangular wire, often with extra torque placed into it prior to overjet correction, and gentle forces. Also, brackets with increased incisor torque (Chapter 3) are beneficial in these situations.

417

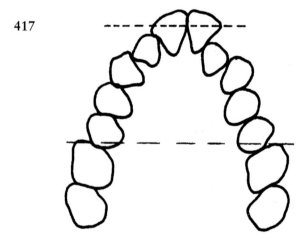

418

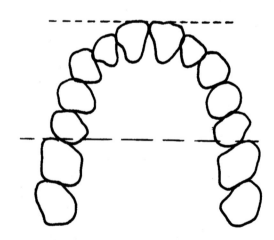

417 This figure shows the starting archform of a typical Class II, division 1 case, with narrowing in the premolar regions and proclination of the upper centrals.

418 This figure shows the planned final archform. In cases like this, the overjet will reduce during progress into rectangular wires during leveling and aligning if molars are controlled and bendbacks carefully used in the early wires, with passive tiebacks in the opening rectangular wires.

Distal movement or limiting forward growth of the maxilla

Assessment of the position of maxillary bone may be measured by the SNA angle favored by Steiner [2] (normal 82°) or by dropping a perpendicular from nasion through Frankfort Plane, and using a normal of 0mm for 'A' point (**419**), as recommended by McNamara.[3] It is important to note that this normal is subjective to an extent and was based on '... a sample of 111 young adults who, in the opinion of my co-workers and myself, have good facial configuration ...' It should be used for guidance only, and not rigidly adhered to.

When it is clear that increased overjet is due to a forward position of maxillary bone, it is appropriate to attempt to use orthopedic headgear forces or Class II elastics (to be discussed later) to influence maxillary growth in the growing individual. As previously stated, this type of movement is not required in a high percentage of cases since most individuals with Class II malocclusions and overjets show normal or retrusive maxillary positions. The distalization of the maxilla itself is difficult and requires good co-operation with heavy orthopaedic forces. Usually such forces to the maxilla will limit its forward growth, which would be approximately 1 mm per year in a growing child.[1]

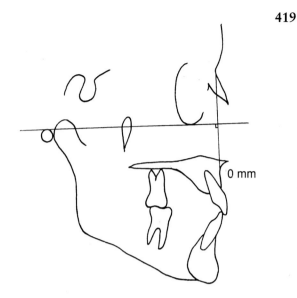

419

419 Normal position of the maxilla, relating 'A' point to a perpendicular from nasion through the Frankfort horizontal plane, as recommended by McNamara.[3]

Mesial movement of the mandible

In addition to helping overjet reduction, mesial movement of the mandible generally produces an improvement in facial harmony and balance in a large percentage of cases with increased overjet. If this can be achieved, then upper incisor retraction can be properly controlled and minimized for the best esthetic results. Figure **420** illustrates the normal position of the mandible in relation to nasion perpendicular. Also, an SNB angle of 80° as recommended by Steiner can be used as a horizontal reference for mandibular position.

The first factor responsible for mesial movement of the mandible is forward mandibular growth rotation. While it is not possible to accurately predict the extent of growth rotation in each individual case, there are general indicators that are helpful in predicting the tendencies towards this growth. Bjork[6] discussed mandibular growth rotation at some length and described two categories: forward rotation and backward rotation.

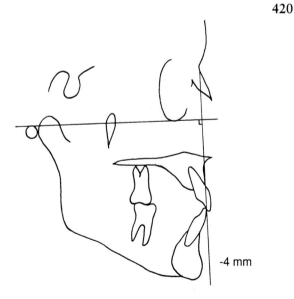

420

420 Normal position of the mandible in relation to nasion perpendicular (McNamara).

147

Forward growth rotation occurs more frequently and is divided into three groups:

- Those with the center of rotation at the temporomandibular joints. This occurs when there is loss of teeth or strong musculature and results in deepening of the bite.
- Those with the center of rotation at the incisal edges of the lower anterior teeth. This occurs when there is marked development of posterior face height and normal increase in anterior face height. In this type of growth the posterior aspect of the mandible rotates away from the maxilla.
- Those with the center of rotation in the premolar area. This can occur when there is no anterior contact. In this type of growth the posterior face height increases, and the anterior face height shows progressive under-development. The result is often a skeletal deep bite.

Backward rotation of the mandible fortunately occurs infrequently and is divided into two groups:

- Those with the center of rotation at the temporomandibular joint. This can occur when the bite is opened by orthodontic therapy and results in an increase in anterior face height.
- Those with the center of rotation at the most distally occluding molar. This occurs due to the sagittal growth direction at the mandibular condyles, and often results in a skeletal open bite.

Figures **421** and **422** show mandibular contours typical of forward and backward mandibular growth rotation. Bjork also found that the average rate of mandibular growth in the male was 3 mm/year with a prepubertal minimum of 1.5 mm/year at age 11.5 and a pubertal maximum of 5.5 mm/year at 14.5 years of age (measured from condyle head to pogonion).

The Michigan growth studies confirm these measurements stating that from the ages of 6 to 16, males experienced an overall increase in mandibular length from 103.0 mm to 133.6 mm, which is an average increase of 3 mm per year. Females experienced an overall increase in mandibular length from 100.5 mm to 123.6 mm from the age of 6 to 16 which is an average increase of 2.3 mm per year.

While there have been claims that functional appliances 'stimulate' mandibular growth beyond a patient's normal growth potential, clinical research does not support this claim. For example, Harvold's studies indicated that the activator appliance brought about an additional increase of 1.0 mm to 1.5 mm in overall mandibular length on average, which was clearly not enough to correct a significant overjet or Class II molar relationship.[7] Harvold stated that the correction of Class II molar relationship with functional appliances was primarily due to limiting the downward and forward eruption of the upper posterior teeth, while allowing for upward and forward eruption of the lower posterior teeth.

421

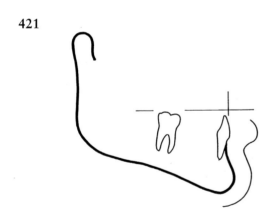

421 Mandibular contour typical of forward growth rotation.

422

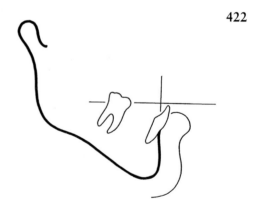

422 Mandibular contour typical of backward growth rotation.

He further stated that overjet reduction occurred primarily as a result of distal tipping of upper incisors and mesial tipping of lower incisors.

Mills[8] reviewed the literature extensively and was also unable to demonstrate any significant increase in mandibular length as a result of functional appliance use. This is not to say that functional appliances cannot be used in the management of Class II cases with overjets, but that their true methods of correction must be appreciated.

The second factor responsible for mesial movement of the mandible is limiting of posterior vertical dental and skeletal development. On a geometric basis, any mechanical procedures which reduce or maintain the MM angle will produce mesial movement of pogonion in the facial profile (**423**) The use of high-pull headgear, palatal bars, lingual arches, and posterior bite plates favors control of this type. Also, the extraction of premolar teeth makes vertical control easier. Use of inter-maxillary elastics in high angle cases, as well as cervical headgear and anterior bite plates tends to open the MM angle and produce unfavorable change in the position of pogonion (**424**). Non-extraction treatment also makes it difficult to prevent the MM angle opening.

In summary, an understanding of the importance of vertical factors listed is essential to proper management of overjet reduction.

MM angle tends to open in response to:

- Non-extraction treatment
- Cervical headgear
- Prolonged intermaxillary elastics
- Anterior bite plates

MM Angle tends to close or be maintained in response to:

- Extraction treatment
- High pull headgears
- Palatal bars and lingual arches
- Posterior bite plates

In Class II division 1 cases with an average or increased MM angle, vertical control is important to reduce the angle, or at least prevent it from increasing. Pogonion will move distally in the profile if the MM angle is allowed to increase, and this unfavorable change will be geometrically greater in higher angle patterns.

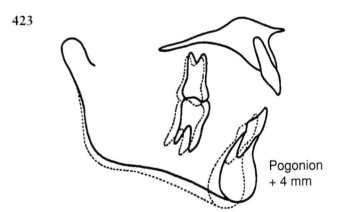

423 The geometrical basis whereby pogonion moves mesially in the profile as MM angle reduces. It is difficult to close the MM angle with routine fixed appliance therapy — maintaining the MM angle is a general indicator of effecting posterior vertical control in high angle cases.

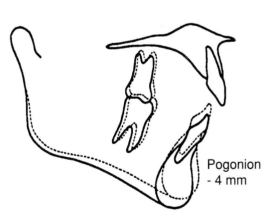

424 The effect of increasing the MM angle on pogonion.

149

The Mechanics of Overjet Reduction

Patients with Class II malocclusion and increased overjet present with a wide variety of skeletal and dental patterns.[5] Horizontally their Class II skeletal patterns may be the result of a protrusive, normal or a retrusive maxilla in combination with a protrusive, normal or retrusive mandible. Occasionally they may demonstrate Class II posterior dental relationships with Class I skeletal patterns. Vertically they may range from high mandibular plane angle cases to low mandibular plane angle cases, from cases with the palatal plane tipped up anteriorly to cases with the palatal plane tipped down anteriorly. Also, there are the asymmetrical variations of Class II cases which are beyond the scope of this text.

Despite these many variations there are only three primary methods used to correct Class II molar relationships and reduce overjets. The primary methods are:

- Class II elastics
- Headgear (Facebows)
- Functional appliances

These three provide the force or energy (and perhaps the release of forces with functional appliances) to correct these malocclusions. Fixed appliances serve primarily to provide tooth alignment as well as attachments for Class II elastics and headgears. A secondary method of overjet reduction involves extraction of upper bicuspids only and retraction of the upper anterior segment.

The three primary methods can be used separately or in combination and ultimately their correct use is the key to a successful result.

CLASS II ELASTICS

Class II elastics (**425**) are used with fixed appliances and have the following effects:

- They move the upper teeth distally.
- They move the lower teeth mesially.
- They posture the mandible forward.
- They cause no significant speech interference.
- They are reasonably esthetic.
- They cause an extrusive force on the lower molars.
- They cause an extrusive force on the upper incisors.

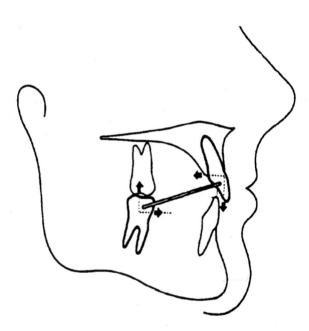

425 The primary force vectors involved in the use of Class II elastics.

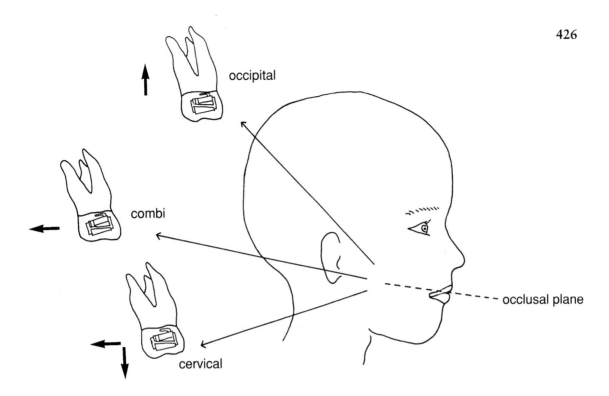

426 Primary vectors of force generated by the use of high-pull, cervical pull and combination high-pull and cervical pull headgears.

HEADGEARS (FACEBOWS)

Headgears (facebows) are used with three main force vectors (high-pull, cervical pull, and combination high-pull/cervical pull, **426**). They can be described as producing the following effects:

- They move the upper first molars distally.
- They allow for accurate vertical forces on upper first molars.
- They produce an orthopedic change on the maxilla.
- They cause no anchorage loss on the lower arch.
- They provide anchorage support for Class III elastics and upper incisor retraction.
- They may cause a distalizing effect on the mandible.[9]
- They are unesthetic and somewhat uncomfortable.

FUNCTIONAL APPLIANCES

Although discussion of functional appliances is beyond the scope of this chapter, the effects of the toothborne varieties such as bionators, can be described as follows:

- They posture the mandible forward.
- They have an orthopedic effect on the maxilla.
- They effect vertical control of the posterior teeth.
- They tip the upper incisors distally.
- They tip the lower incisors mesially.
- They must be held in position by the patient.
- They affect speech and esthetics.

Clinical Examples

Decisions concerning the methods of overjet reduction must be made at the initial case diagnosis so this stage of treatment can be carried out in the easiest and most efficient manner with the best possible end results. When deciding the overjet reduction mechanics for an individual case, it is essential to have a clear idea of the vertical and horizontal position of the maxilla and mandible, as well as the positions of the posterior dental segments and the upper and lower incisors. Just prior to overjet reduction, a progress lateral skull X-ray is helpful in re-evaluating initial treatment objectives, but experienced orthodontists may feel that in many cases it is possible to make a clinical judgement, without the use of a progress X-ray. This is then followed by the use of one or more of the above described methods of Class II molar correction and overjet reduction.

A series of extraction and non-extraction examples will now be presented showing various clinical situations, followed by a discussion of treatment needs for each case. In the examples, an ideal position of lower incisors of APo + 2 mm has been used, although the authors accept that other clinicians may wish to use alternative assessment methods or normals. The effectiveness of the recommended mechanics remains undiminished when using different normals.

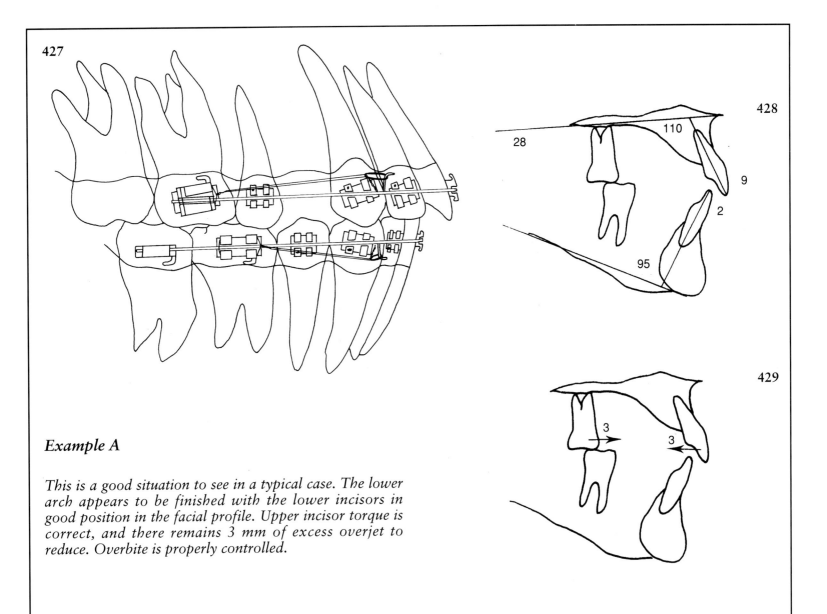

427

428

28
110
9
2
95

429

3 →
← 3

Example A

This is a good situation to see in a typical case. The lower arch appears to be finished with the lower incisors in good position in the facial profile. Upper incisor torque is correct, and there remains 3 mm of excess overjet to reduce. Overbite is properly controlled.

Treatment Needs:

The remaining 6 mm of upper space may be closed by reciprocal space closure, using sliding mechanics, because molar relationship is slightly Class III. The molars and premolars will move mesially by 3 mm as the canines and incisors move distally by the same amount. Night-time headgear support could be used if the molars moved forwards more rapidly than anticipated.

The rectangular wire will allow bodily control of the upper incisors, provided force levels are light, and provided the upper incisor brackets recommended in Chapter 3 are used. Ideally, upper second molars should have been included in the hook-up, as palatal cusps will tend to drop down as they follow the upper first molars mesially.

A passive tieback is placed to hold lower space closed. An active tieback, with a module on the soldered archwire hook delivers space closure force in the upper arch, which will simultaneously reduce the overjet.

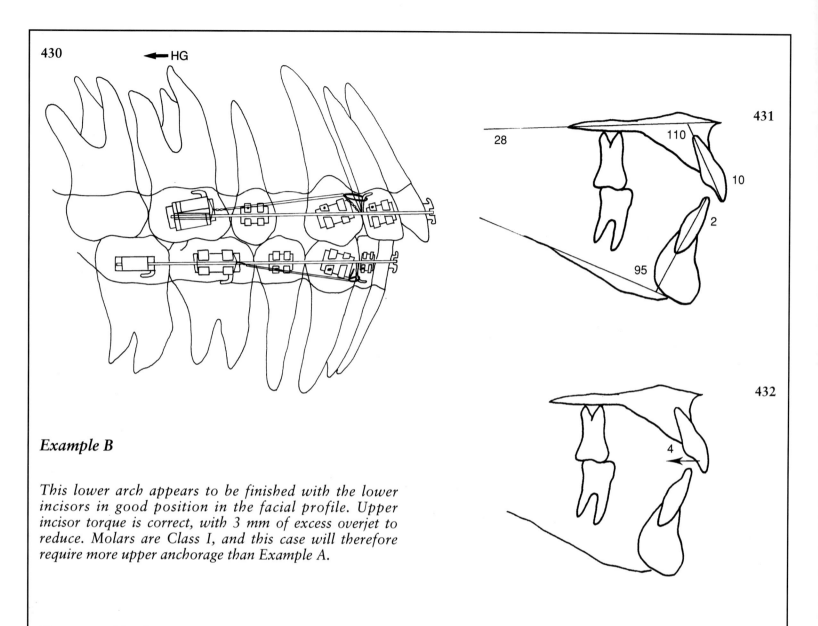

430   ← HG

431

28   110   10   2   95

432

4

Example B

This lower arch appears to be finished with the lower incisors in good position in the facial profile. Upper incisor torque is correct, with 3 mm of excess overjet to reduce. Molars are Class I, and this case will therefore require more upper anchorage than Example A.

Treatment Needs

The remaining upper space may not be closed by reciprocal space closure, because molar relationship is Class I. It will deteriorate into a Class II relationship without some form of support, because the molars and premolars will tend to move mesially by 3 mm as the canines and incisors move distally. Support from a sleeping headgear and/or a palatal bar will be needed to protect the molar relationship during overjet reduction.

Upper second molars would normally be banded for proper torque control. The rectangular wire will allow bodily control of the upper incisors, provided force levels are light, and provided the upper incisor brackets recommended in Chapter 3 are used. A passive tieback is placed to hold lower space closed. An active upper tieback, with a module on the soldered archwire hook delivers space closure force in the upper arch, which will reduce the overjet.

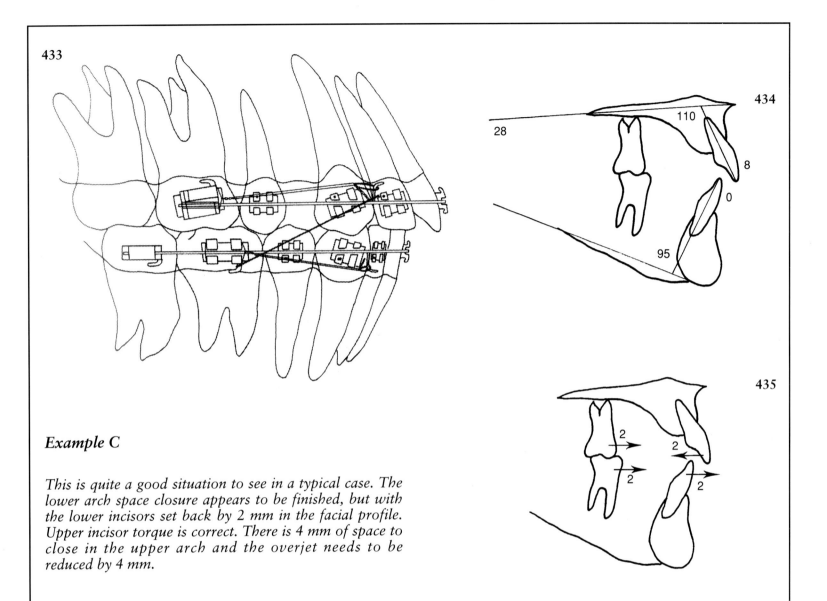

433

434

28

110

8

0

95

435

2

2

2

2

Example C

This is quite a good situation to see in a typical case. The lower arch space closure appears to be finished, but with the lower incisors set back by 2 mm in the facial profile. Upper incisor torque is correct. There is 4 mm of space to close in the upper arch and the overjet needs to be reduced by 4 mm.

Treatment Needs

The remaining upper space may be closed by reciprocal space closure, with some support from Class II elastics which will protect the molar relationship by bringing the lower arch forward to a position close to APo + 2 mm. In the upper arch the molars and premolars will move mesially 2 mm as the canines and incisors move distally 2 mm. In this case the MM angle is 28° (average) and Class II elastics may routinely be used in these average or lower angle cases. Intermaxillary elastics may be contra-indicated in higher angle patterns, but in these cases, the lower incisors are seldom found to be behind APo line at this stage. A high pull headgear is normally preferred for upper molar support during overjet reduction in higher angle cases.

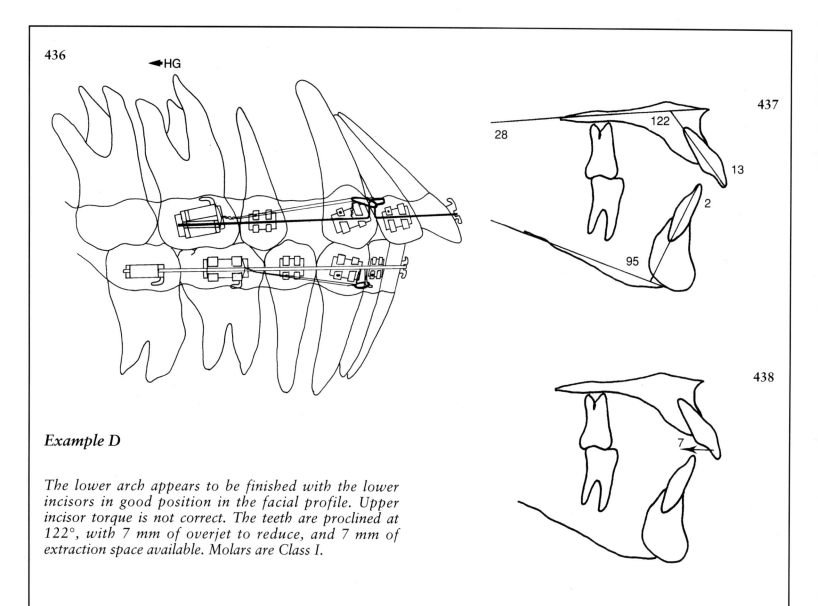

436 HG

437 28 122 13 2 95

438 7

Example D

The lower arch appears to be finished with the lower incisors in good position in the facial profile. Upper incisor torque is not correct. The teeth are proclined at 122°, with 7 mm of overjet to reduce, and 7 mm of extraction space available. Molars are Class I.

Treatment Needs

The remaining upper space may not be closed by reciprocal space closure, because upper molars and premolars will move mesially as the canines and incisors move distally, and the Class I molar relationship will thus be lost. The drawing shows a round wire being used, because approximately 10° of tipping is permissible, but a rectangular wire will allow better bodily control of the upper incisors, provided force levels are light.

If a large overjet needs to be reduced in this way, brackets with additional torque as recommended in Chapter 3 would be required for the incisors, and rectangular wire would be essential. Support from a sleeping headgear and/or a palatal bar would definitely be needed, although proclined incisors generally require less anchorage in the early stages of overjet reduction, whether round or rectangular wires are used, because initial movement is tipping.

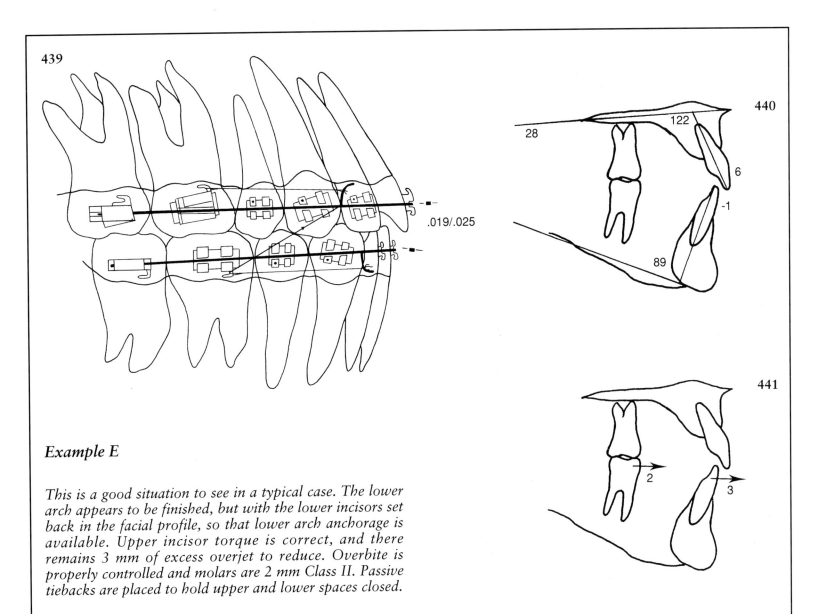

439

.019/.025

440

28

122

6

-1

89

441

2

3

Example E

This is a good situation to see in a typical case. The lower arch appears to be finished, but with the lower incisors set back in the facial profile, so that lower arch anchorage is available. Upper incisor torque is correct, and there remains 3 mm of excess overjet to reduce. Overbite is properly controlled and molars are 2 mm Class II. Passive tiebacks are placed to hold upper and lower spaces closed.

Treatment Needs

The 3 mm of overjet may be reduced using Class II elastic traction, as the MM angle is at an average figure of 28°. The upper arch can act as an anchorage unit with teeth ligated to a rectangular wire. The lower incisors are at 89° and can therefore be allowed to tip forwards by up to 6° in this case. As the overjet reduces and the lower teeth move mesially in the profile the molars will move towards a Class I relationship.

The tips of the lower incisors can be expected to move mesially more than the lower molars do (3 mm compared with 2 mm), because part of the incisor change involves tipping. The lower rectangular wire can carry a little labial crown torque in the incisor region, to assist forward tipping of incisors. The upper rectangular wire allows bodily control of the upper incisors, provided force levels are light.

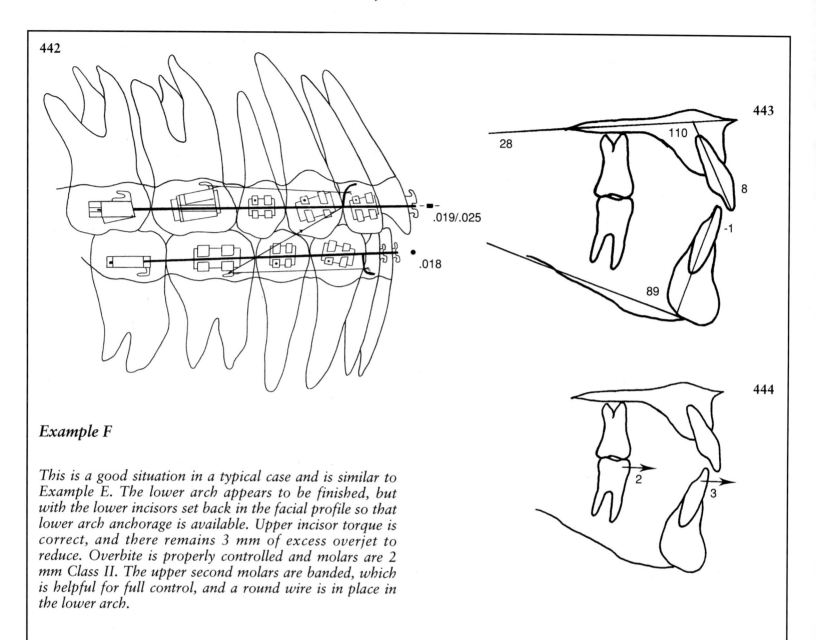

442

.019/.025

.018

443

28
110
8
-1
89

444

2
3

Example F

This is a good situation in a typical case and is similar to Example E. The lower arch appears to be finished, but with the lower incisors set back in the facial profile so that lower arch anchorage is available. Upper incisor torque is correct, and there remains 3 mm of excess overjet to reduce. Overbite is properly controlled and molars are 2 mm Class II. The upper second molars are banded, which is helpful for full control, and a round wire is in place in the lower arch.

Treatment Needs

The 3 mm of overjet may be reduced using Class II elastic traction, as the MM angle is at an average figure of 28°. The upper arch can provide anchorage with teeth ligated to a rectangular wire. The lower incisors are at 89° and round wire can therefore be used for initial overjet reduction, allowing lower incisors to tip forwards by up to 6° in this case. If the overjet was larger, then a lower rectangular wire would be preferable to a round one, to maximize the available lower anchorage potential. As the overjet reduces, and the lower teeth move mesially in the profile, the molars will become Class I. The tips of the lower incisors can be expected to move mesially more than the lower molars do, because part of the incisor change would involve tipping.

Upper second molars have been included in the hook-up to ensure proper control of palatal cusps. Passive tiebacks are placed to hold upper and lower spaces closed. Later in treatment, rectangular wire will be essential in the lower arch, to complete detailing and finishing.

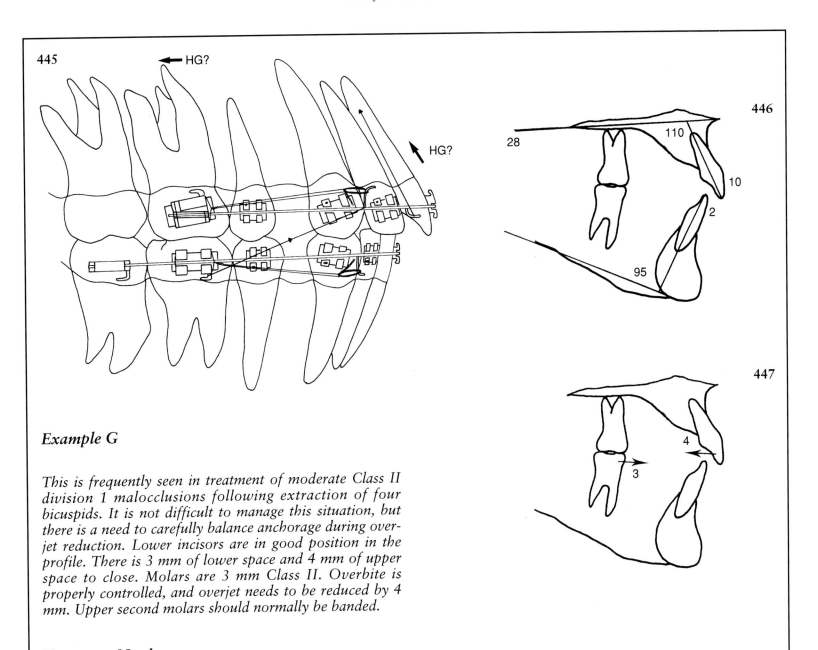

445 HG?

HG?

446

28   110

10

2

95

447

4

3

Example G

This is frequently seen in treatment of moderate Class II division 1 malocclusions following extraction of four bicuspids. It is not difficult to manage this situation, but there is a need to carefully balance anchorage during overjet reduction. Lower incisors are in good position in the profile. There is 3 mm of lower space and 4 mm of upper space to close. Molars are 3 mm Class II. Overbite is properly controlled, and overjet needs to be reduced by 4 mm. Upper second molars should normally be banded.

Treatment Needs

This case shows the ease and sophistication of sliding mechanics and group movement of teeth. The 4 mm of overjet may be reduced with support from Class II elastic traction, as the MM angle is at an average figure of 28°. Sleeping headgear will be necessary to upper molars (or possibly to the upper archwire anteriorly, if there is a gummy smile tendency).

The Class II elastics will change the balance of lower arch space closure. It will not be reciprocal; lower molars and premolars will move mesially and lower incisors will tend not to move distally. The headgear support to the upper arch will ensure that the upper labial segment moves distally by the necessary 4 mm, while upper molars are supported and prevented from moving mesially. Month-by-month monitoring will be needed, and good co-operation will be needed from the patient, but little work is required from the orthodontist. Ideally, upper second molars should have been included in the hook-up.

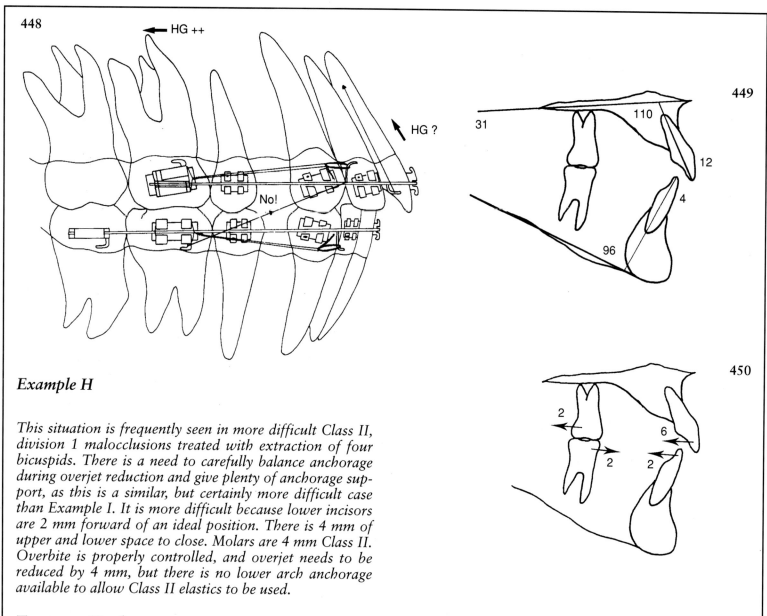

Example H

This situation is frequently seen in more difficult Class II, division 1 malocclusions treated with extraction of four bicuspids. There is a need to carefully balance anchorage during overjet reduction and give plenty of anchorage support, as this is a similar, but certainly more difficult case than Example I. It is more difficult because lower incisors are 2 mm forward of an ideal position. There is 4 mm of upper and lower space to close. Molars are 4 mm Class II. Overbite is properly controlled, and overjet needs to be reduced by 4 mm, but there is no lower arch anchorage available to allow Class II elastics to be used.

Treatment Needs

The 4 mm of overjet must not be reduced using support from Class II elastics, as the lower incisors will be brought even further forward in the profile. Good co-operation will be essential, as considerable headgear wear will be necessary to the upper arch. The headgear support to the upper arch will ensure that the upper labial segment moves distally by the necessary 6 mm. Lower space closure will need to be reciprocal, with molars travelling mesially by 2 mm and incisors going distally by the same amount. Treatment response will generally be better in the growing patient rather than the non-growing adult, as it is difficult to achieve correction of this type only with tooth movement. The rectangular wire will allow bodily control of the upper incisors, provided force levels are light. Ideally, upper second molars should have been included in the hook-up.

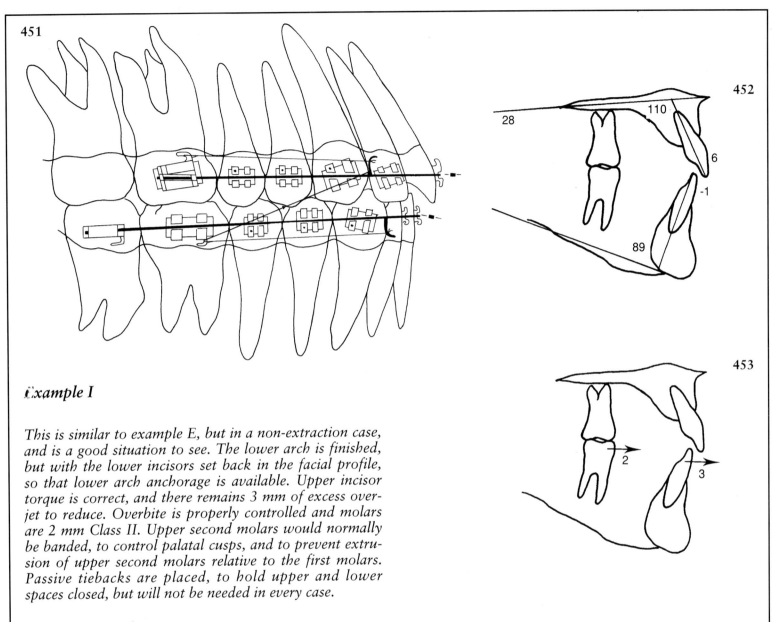

451

452

453

Example I

This is similar to example E, but in a non-extraction case, and is a good situation to see. The lower arch is finished, but with the lower incisors set back in the facial profile, so that lower arch anchorage is available. Upper incisor torque is correct, and there remains 3 mm of excess overjet to reduce. Overbite is properly controlled and molars are 2 mm Class II. Upper second molars would normally be banded, to control palatal cusps, and to prevent extrusion of upper second molars relative to the first molars. Passive tiebacks are placed, to hold upper and lower spaces closed, but will not be needed in every case.

Treatment Needs

The 3 mm overjet may be reduced using Class II elastic traction, as the MM angle is at an average figure of 28°. If the angle is average or below average, Class II mechanics can be used to reduce an overjet in a case like this, but in higher angle patterns such elastic use should be minimal to avoid further opening of the angle. The lower incisors are at 89° and can therefore be allowed to tip forwards by up to 6° in this case.

The upper arch can act as an anchorage unit with teeth ligated to a rectangular wire. As the overjet reduces, and the lower teeth move mesially in the profile, the molar relationship will improve towards Class I. The tips of the lower incisors can be expected to move mesially rather more than the lower molars do, because part of the incisor change involves tipping. Patients with teeth in this arrangement will tend to posture the mandible into a forward position, to obtain a convenient Class I dental occlusion, and good intercuspation, but with the condyles forward in the fossae. Care is therefore needed to ensure that the overjet has been properly reduced.

454

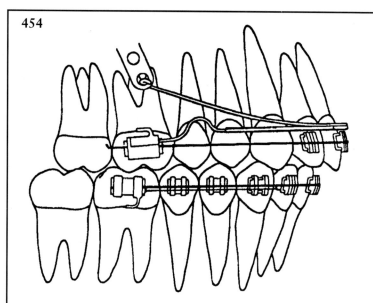

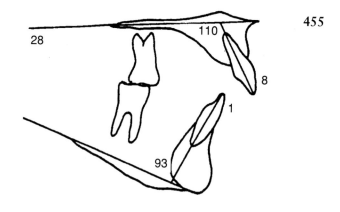

455

Example J

This case requires the greatest care and management of any of the three non-extraction cases presented. The patient initially showed a Class II, division I malocclusion with a full Class II molar relationship and an 8 mm overjet. The initial stage of treatment involves leveling and aligning the lower arch to a rectangular wire, while initiating Class II molar correction with a combination high-pull/cervical facebow headgear to the first molars. The upper incisors are bracketed for alignment and bite opening.

The overbite is corrected as a result of upper incisor control and leveling the lower arch to a rectangular wire. The lower incisors are I mm in front of APo after leveling, and can only be slightly advanced during overjet reduc-

tion. The upper incisors show adequate torque, and the patient continues to demonstrate an overjet of 8 mm.

The patient has not worn the headgear consistently, and the molars remain 6 mm in a Class II position. Extraction of upper second molars allows for more effective distalization of the upper first molar. The third molar is then allowed to erupt into the second molar position.

Therefore, in the early stages of treatment, because of the severity of the Class II molar problem an attempt was made to stabilize the lower arch and begin correcting the Class II molar relationship, leaving the overjet reduction for a later stage of treatment. Correction of a severe problem of this type will be easier in a patient showing favorable growth.

Treatment needs

Since the lower incisors are in a nearly ideal position, the remainder of treatment was carried out with the following procedures, beginning with the completion of Class II molar correction:

- The headgear needs to be worn to the upper arch approximately 14 hours per day, usually when the patient is at home and while sleeping (456).
- The patient is then asked to use Class II elastics to an upper sliding jig approximately 10 hours per day (457), with the effect depicted in 458.

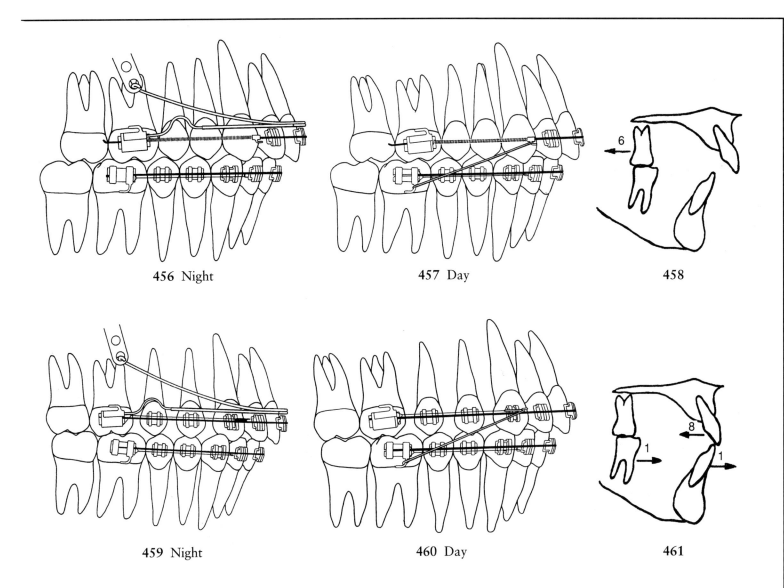

456 Night

457 Day

458

459 Night

460 Day

461

As Andrews has discussed with his 10 hour force theory,[10] the 10 hours of Class II elastics applied to a stabilized and tied back lower arch creates a very minimal drain on lower arch anchorage. Once Class I molar relationship is achieved, overjet reduction is carried out as follows:

- The upper cuspids and bicuspids are bracketed and the upper arch is releveled with continued headgear support.
- The headgear continues to be worn 14 hours per day and the upper arch is tied back in normal fashion to initiate overjet reduction (**459**). During daytime hours approximately 10 hours of Class II elastics are worn to the hooks on the archwire rather than to the sliding jig to complete overjet reduction (**460**), with the effect depicted in **461**.

Therefore, in both these phases of treatment a 24-hour force is applied to the upper arch to first complete molar correction, and then to complete overjet reduction. However, only an intermittent force of 10 hours per day is applied to the lower arch with Class II elastics.

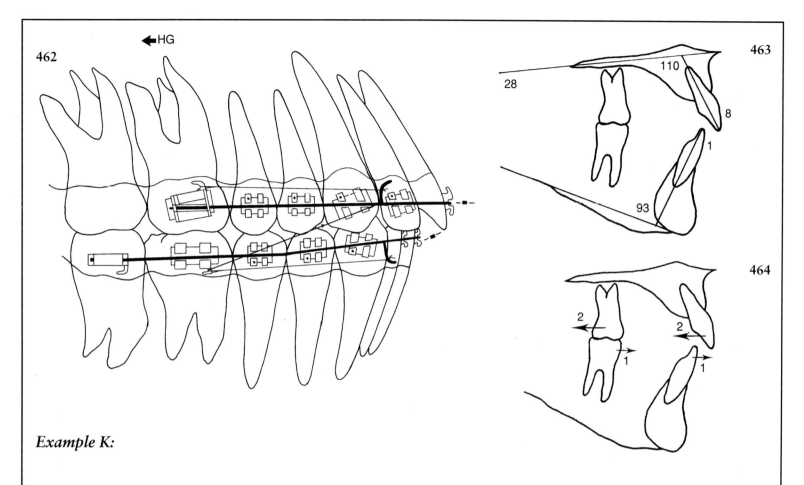

Example K:

This non-extraction case requires careful management and good patient co-operation for proper overjet reduction. The lower arch appears to be finished with the lower incisors almost in correct position in the facial profile, so that very little arch anchorage is available. Lower incisors can only be permitted to move mesially in the profile by 1 mm. Upper incisor torque is correct, and there remains 3 mm of excess overjet to reduce. Overbite is properly controlled (important in this case) and molars are 3 mm Class II. Patients with teeth in this position may tend to posture the mandible forward to achieve a Class I dental relationship, with condyles slightly forward in the fossae.

Treatment Needs

Only a limited amount of Class II elastic traction may be used to reduce the overjet, and therefore headgear support to the upper first molars will be essential. A regime of sleeping headgear, with Class II elastics during the daytime, could be considered. This will give a 24 hour distalizing force on the upper arch and only a 12–14 hour mesializing force on the lower arch.

The lower rectangular wire has additional lingual crown torque in the incisor region to resist forward tipping movement of the incisors. Lower teeth should be ligated hard, so that the lower arch becomes an anchorage unit. Treatment response will generally be better in the growing patient rather than the non-growing adult, as it is difficult to achieve correction in this type of problem only by tooth movement. The rectangular wire will allow bodily control of the upper incisors, provided force levels are light. Ideally, upper second molars should have been included in the hookup.

CASE REPORT JS

A Class II division 1 non-extraction case

A 12 year old boy demonstrating a Class II division 1 mal-occlusion with slight crowding in the lower arch and more severe crowding in the upper arch.

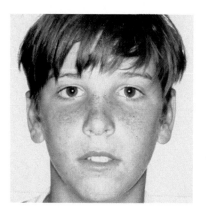

465

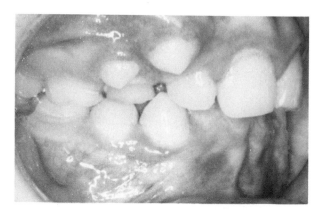

468

Occlusal views show mild lower crowding and more severe upper crowding, with upper canines erupting buccally due to lack of space.

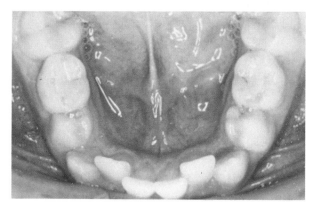

471

466

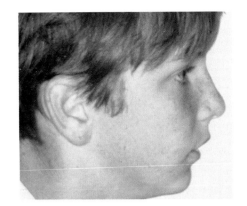

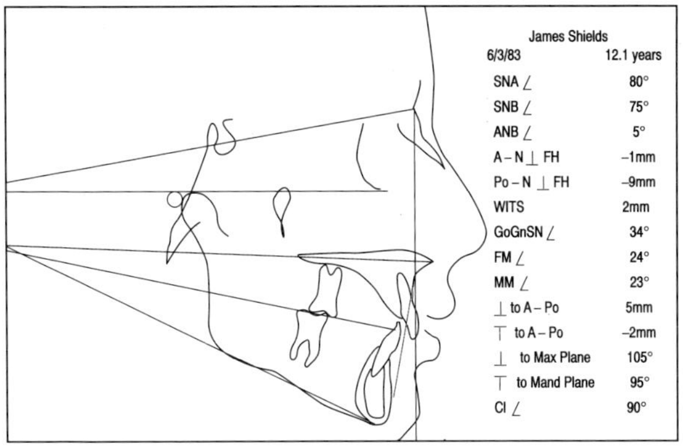

467

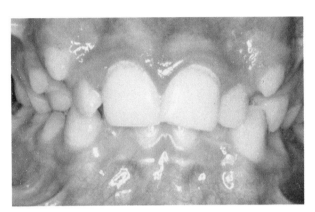

James Shields

6/3/83	12.1 years
SNA ∠	80°
SNB ∠	75°
ANB ∠	5°
A – N ⊥ FH	–1mm
Po – N ⊥ FH	–9mm
WITS	2mm
GoGnSN ∠	34°
FM ∠	24°
MM ∠	23°
⊥ to A – Po	5mm
⊤ to A – Po	–2mm
⊥ to Max Plane	105°
⊤ to Mand Plane	95°
Cl ∠	90°

469

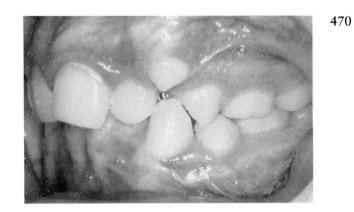

470

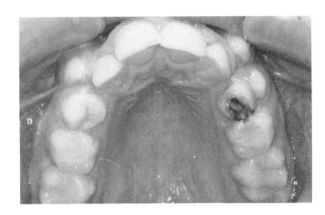

472

The patient was treated using alternating headgear and Class II elastics to a sliding jig during the initial stages of treatment, to correct the molar relationship. The sliding jig consisted of a .020 round wire and a closed coil spring in front of the molar, with a sliding hook in front of the closed coil spring; 473, 474 and 475 show the night-time arrangement.

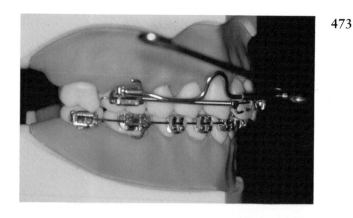

473

A Class II elastic was worn to the sliding hook during daytime hours and the headgear was worn when the patient was at home; 476, 477 and 478 show the daytime arrangement.

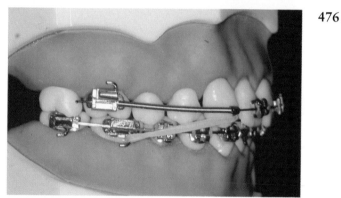

476

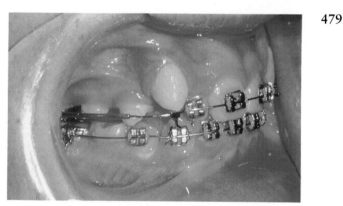

479

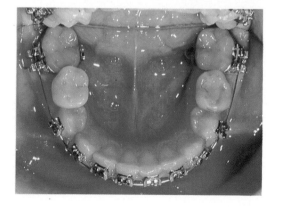

482

474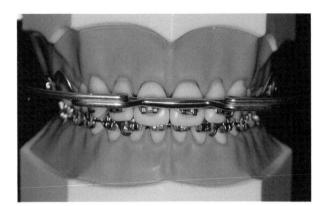

475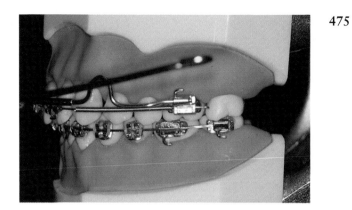

477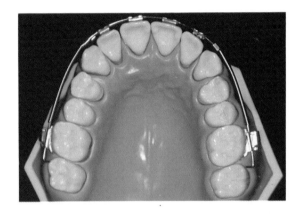

478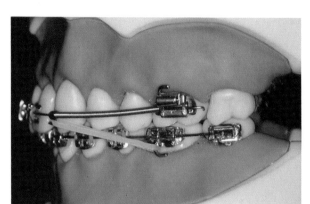

480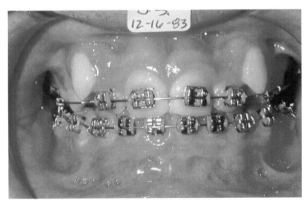

481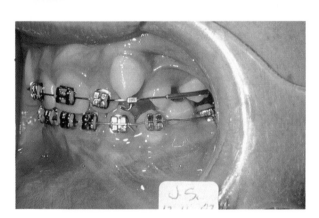

483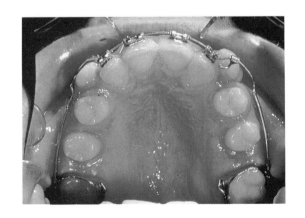

When the molars were in a Class I relationship, the upper premolars and canines were banded and the overjet reduction was completed, using night-time headgear and Class II elastics to the hooks on the rectangular archwires.

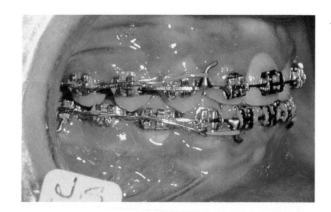

484

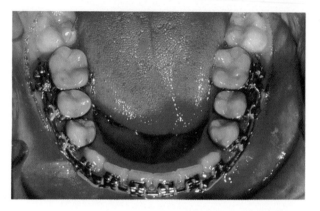

487

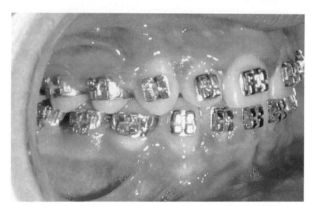

489

485

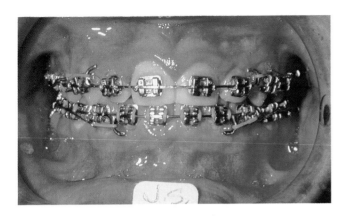

486

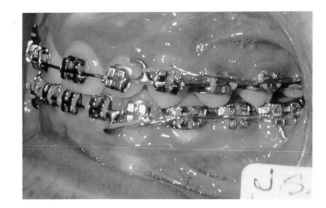

488

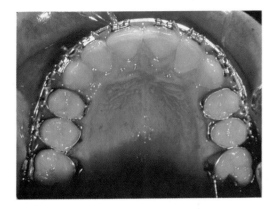

490

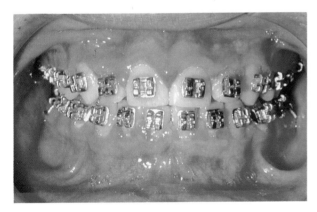

491

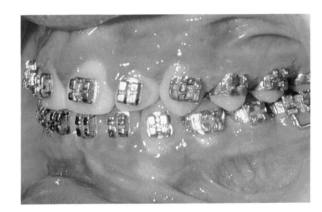

A lower premolar-to-premolar retainer was cemented in place and the patient was asked to wear a nocturnal removable Hawley retainer.

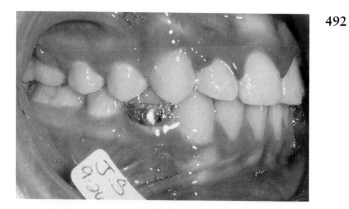

492

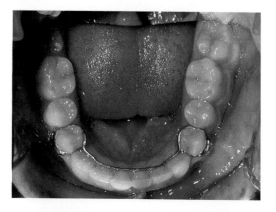

495

The result of non-extraction treatment was a pleasing facial profile, compared with starting profile (**501**).

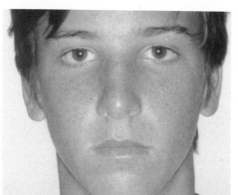

497

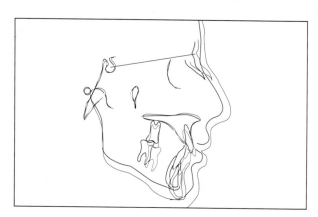

500

493

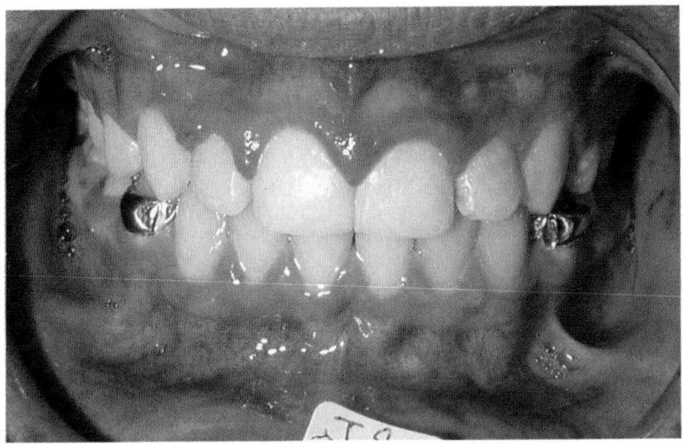

494

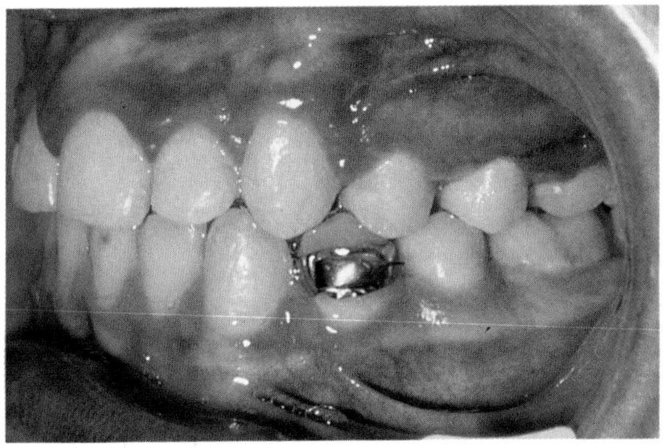

496

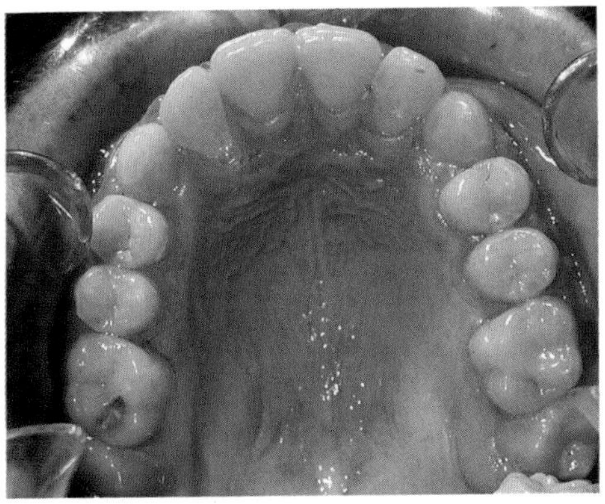

498

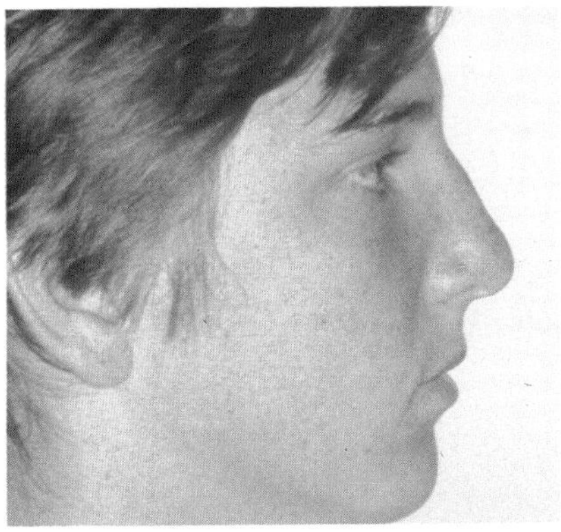

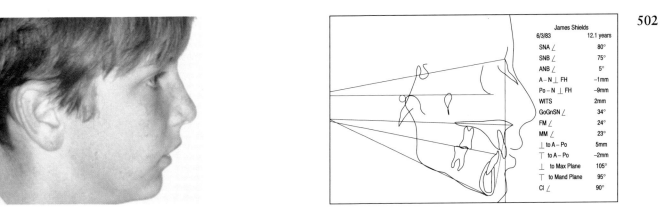

499

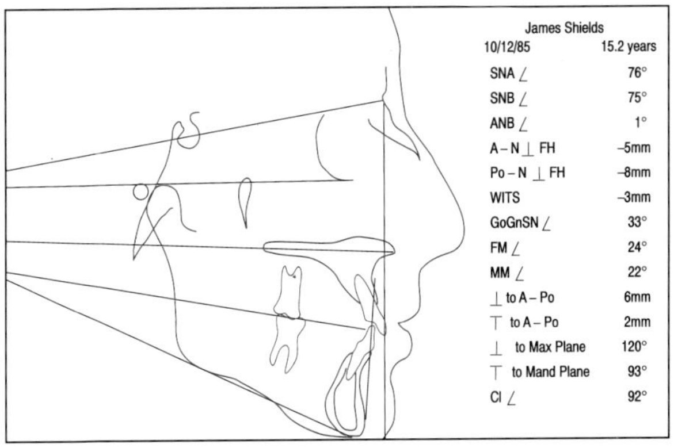

James Shields	
10/12/85	15.2 years
SNA ∠	76°
SNB ∠	75°
ANB ∠	1°
A – N ⊥ FH	–5mm
Po – N ⊥ FH	–8mm
WITS	–3mm
GoGnSN ∠	33°
FM ∠	24°
MM ∠	22°
⊥ to A – Po	6mm
T to A – Po	2mm
⊥ to Max Plane	120°
T to Mand Plane	93°
CI ∠	92°

501

502

James Shields	
6/3/83	12.1 years
SNA ∠	80°
SNB ∠	75°
ANB ∠	5°
A – N ⊥ FH	–1mm
Po – N ⊥ FH	–9mm
WITS	2mm
GoGnSN ∠	34°
FM ∠	24°
MM ∠	23°
⊥ to A – Po	5mm
T to A – Po	–2mm
⊥ to Max Plane	105°
T to Mand Plane	95°
CI ∠	90°

CASE REPORT CG

A Class II division 2 case

A thirteen and a half year old boy with a typical Class II division 2 malocclusion. Upper and lower incisors are retroclined on a low angle pattern.

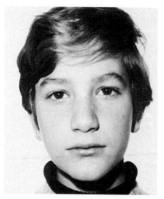

503

Upper lateral incisors show typical rotations and there is a deep, traumatic overbite.

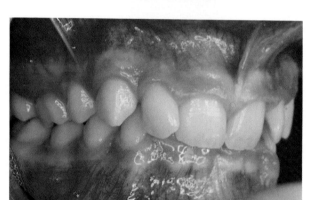

506

A .015 multistrand wire was used to commence upper arch leveling and aligning. Lower anteriors were not bracketed at the start of treatment, because of the overbite.

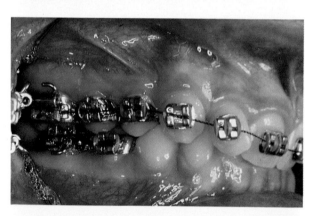

509

After four months of treatment, upper arch leveling was almost complete and the case had a small overjet, with the appearance of a Class II division 1 malocclusion.

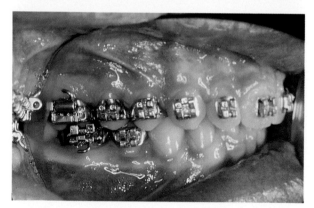

512

504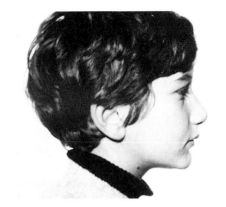

505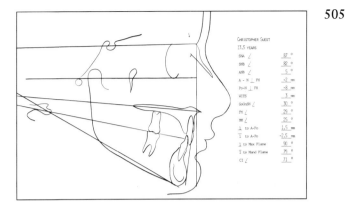

CHRISTOPHER GUEST
13.5 YEARS

SNA ∠	87	°
SNB ∠	82	°
ANB ∠	5	°
A - N ⊥ FH	-2	mm
Po-N ⊥ FH	-8	mm
WITS	3	mm
GoGnSN ∠	30	°
FM ∠	29	°
MM ∠	25	°
1̄ to A-Po	1.5	mm
1̲ to A-Po	-2.5	mm
1̄ to Max Plane	90	°
1̲ to Mand Plane	75	°
CI ∠	71	°

507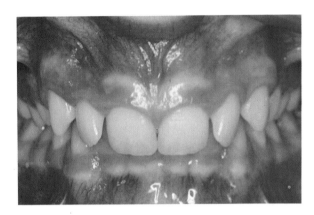

508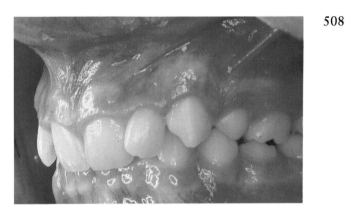

510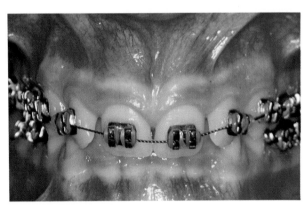

511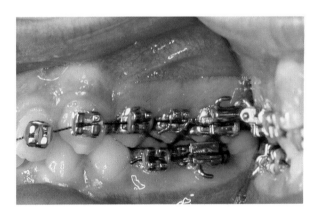

513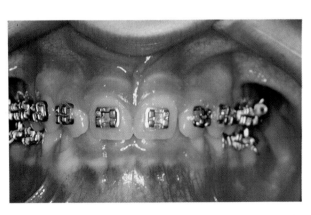

514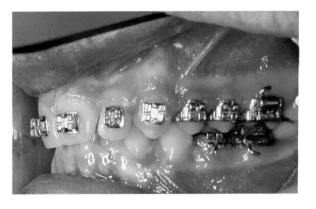

Lower arch leveling and aligning was commenced using light wires, and lower second molars were banded to assist overbite control. An upper rectangular .019/.025 wire was used to torque the upper incisors. Tiebacks were necessary to prevent space opening in the upper arch.

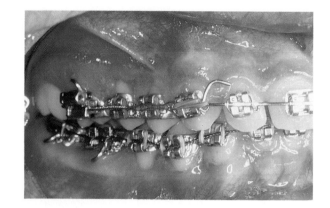

515

With a .016 Australian round wire in the lower arch, light Class II elastics were used to assist overbite control and to commence overjet reduction.

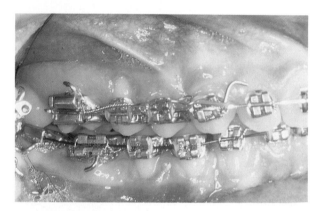

518

Rotation wedges were used to correct the upper lateral incisors.

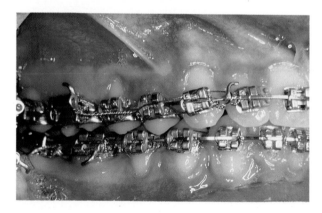

521

516
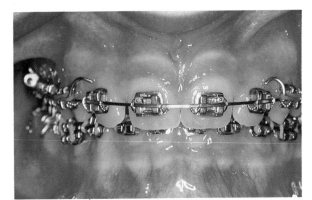

517
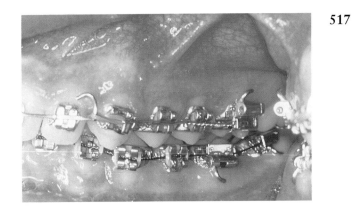

519
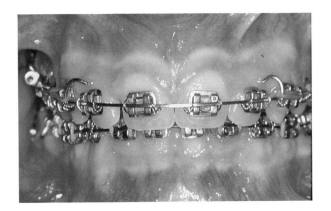

520
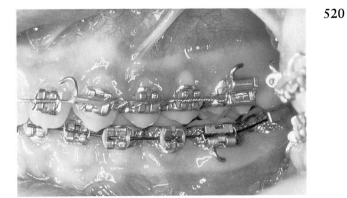

522
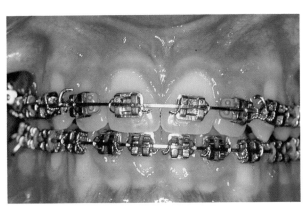

523
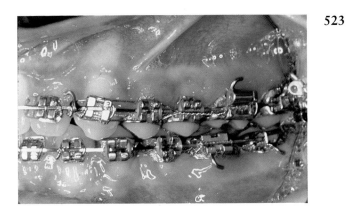

No headgear was used in the treatment of this case. Wedges were maintained on upper lateral incisors until removal of appliances after 18 months of active treatment.

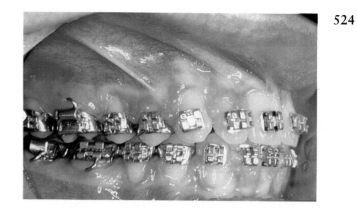

524

The patient was asked to wear removable upper and lower nocturnal acrylic retainers.

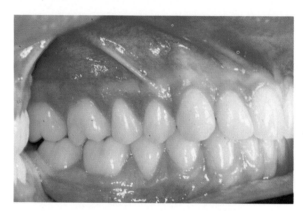

527

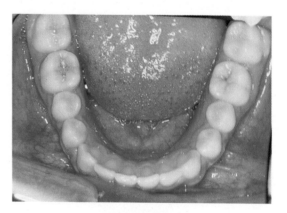

530

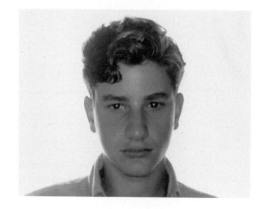

532

525
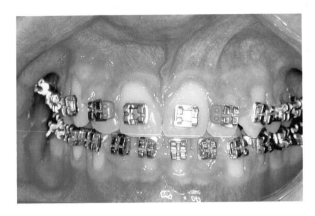

526
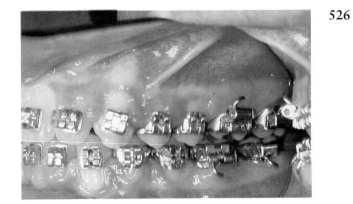

528
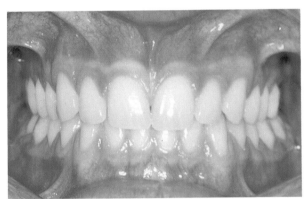

529
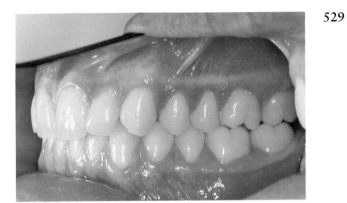

531
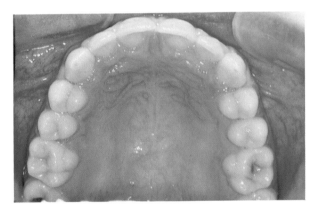

533
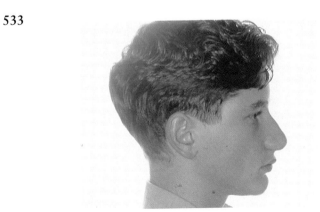

534
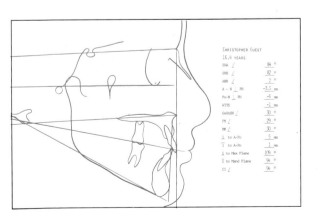

10. SPACE CLOSURE PROCEDURES

Introduction

Following Lawrence F. Andrews' original development of the concept of a Straight-Wire® Appliance, it was reported in 1986 that preadjusted appliance systems in general were used more than twice as much as any other appliance system in the USA.[1, 2] This change brought the possibility, as well as the need, for orthodontists to change their treatment mechanics. In Chapters 2 and 6 the authors have outlined mechanics which have proved effective during the six stages of orthodontic treatment.

The purpose of this chapter is to describe space closure in more detail. It gives important details about the mechanics of space closure, including force levels and the effects of excess force. It reviews possible obstacles to space closure, and describes useful clinical methods of varying anchorage balance, in day-to-day practice.

It has become accepted that extraction of four premolar teeth is necessary for the proper management of some malocclusions. Typically, the 7 mm space in each quadrant has been used by orthodontists to benefit the patient in one or more of three ways:

- Relief of crowding
- Retraction of incisors
- Mesial movement of molars

Prior to treatment, orthodontists plan allocation of space into these three possible uses, and the term 'anchorage control' has been used to describe the manœuvres followed to ensure correct use of space, after elective extraction of healthy teeth.

In Chapter 6 the authors pointed out that the most significant difference between standard edgewise mechanics and mechanics with preadjusted appliances has been observed during space closure. Orthodontists have been able to abandon closing loops, and enjoy the advantage of sliding mechanics, because of level slot line-up. This has freed them from the need to monitor individual tooth movements, and hence allowed them to give greater attention to facial profile considerations.

Treatment Mechanics during Space Closure

A working rectangular archwire size of .019/.025 has proved to be the most effective in a .022 slot preadjusted system. Larger wires, although more rigid, restricted free sliding. Round wires and smaller rectangular wire sizes were evaluated, as possible alternatives, but were found to give less precise control of torque and overbite. Hooks, made of 0.6 mm stainless steel or 0.7 mm brass, were soldered to upper and lower archwires in the positions shown in 535. The average dimensions of 38 mm and 26 mm fitted more than 50% of clinical requirements, and wires were pre-fabricated to this size. Additional sizes of 35 mm and 41 mm (upper) and 24 mm and 28 mm (lower) were found to cover most instances where average hook sizes were not appropriate.

To produce space closure, force was delivered by elastic tiebacks (537, 538). With the elastic module stretched by 2–3 mm (or to twice its unstretched dimension) they have been found to consistently deliver approximately 1 mm of space closure per month, providing no inhibitors were present, as described later. It is advisable to stretch or 'work' the elastic module on the cane prior to activation, to achieve the desired force level (see 28). Typically, space closed more easily in high angle patterns, with soft musculature, than in lower angle patterns. Alternative force delivery systems were evaluated and all had disadvantages. An elastic module chain gave variable force, was difficult to keep clean, and sometimes fell off. Elastic bands, applied by the patient and changed daily, were not consistent because of co-operation factors. Stainless steel coils, of 'Pletcher' type, were found to

535

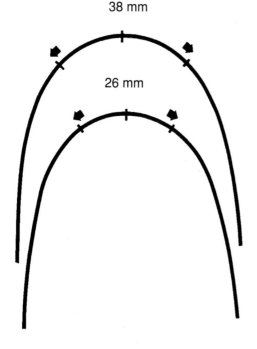

38 mm

26 mm

535 Upper and lower archwires with most frequently used hook positions. The arch-form has been used by the authors for more than eight years and has proved appropriate in more than 80% of clinical situations, when using preadjusted brackets. Most frequently used hook sizes were:
    Upper 35 mm, 38 mm and 41 mm
    Lower 24 mm, 26 mm and 28 mm.

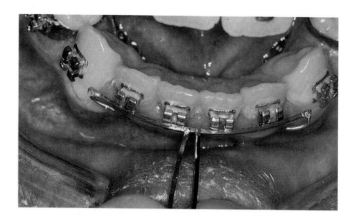

536

536 A simple gauge can be constructed to measure hook positions for each case.

deliver excess force and to be unhygienic. Four possible methods of attaching hooks to rectangular wire can be considered:

- Rectangular Tru-Arch™ wires can be purchased from the manufacturers, with two brass hooks soldered in place at the factory.
- Brass wire hooks can be hand soldered with an electro soldering system, using 0.7 mm or 0.8 mm (.028 or .032 inch) brass wire disposable electrodes. Ball electrodes of a medium size from Ormco (Ref. 758-0233) have proved the most useful.
- Soft stainless steel 0.6 mm (.024 inch) wire can be carefully tack welded in the hook positions and then soldered with a flame, using solder paste, taking care to avoid overheating the base wire.
- Crimpable hooks can be squeezed onto the rectangular wire, after marking positions with a marker pencil. Care is needed to fully crimp the hooks, to avoid them sliding along the wire and retracting canines!

Generally the authors favor methods 1, 2 or 3, and do not currently use crimpable hooks. It is possible to make up a simple gauge to estimate hook positions for a particular case.

One millimetre or more space closure was routinely achieved each month, using the recommended mechanics, and replacing the tiebacks every 4–6 weeks. It was found possible to increase the rate of space closure, particularly in higher angle patterns, by raising the force a little, using thinner archwires, or by applying lingual or palatal forces, either coincidentally or in an alternating routine with buccal forces. Unwanted changes were found to accompany this more rapid rate of space closure. These included loss of control in terms of torque, rotation, and tip, with evidence of excessive soft tissue build-up in the extraction sites.

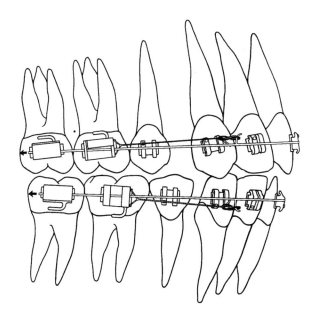

537

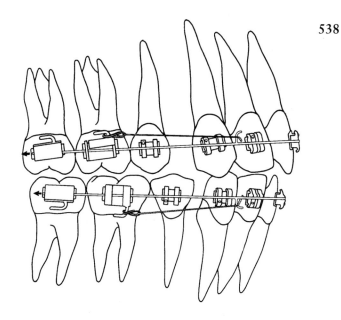

538

537, 538 Elastic tiebacks delivering 50–150 Gms of space closure force. Group movement and sliding mechanics were combined for gentle, controlled space closure. Approximately 0.5 mm of incisor retraction and 0.5 mm of mesial molar movement normally occurred during a month.

The Efficiency of Elastic Module Tiebacks compared with Nickel Titanium Springs

539

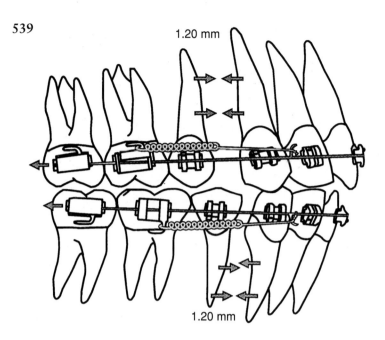

539 Nickel titanium springs delivered approximately 1.20 mm per month of space closure.

During 1991 Samuels, Rudge and Mair compared the rate of space closure using elastic modules and nickel titanium springs.[3] They analyzed tooth movement in 17 subjects using study models. All the cases involved extraction of four first premolars, and Straight-Wire Appliance® brackets were used, with .022 slot size. Archwires were .019/.025 stainless steel, and were in place for at least one month before space closure was commenced. The springs were closed coil medium grade (yellow) Sentalloy™ by GAC, as superelastic nickel titanium has been described as producing a light continuous force over a long range of action.[4]

They found the rate of space closure was significantly greater and more consistent with nickel titanium closed coil springs (539) than with elastic modules (540). The coil springs delivered approximately 1.20 mm per month compared with 0.76 mm per month from the modules. The rate of space closure is compared in the graph (541).

540

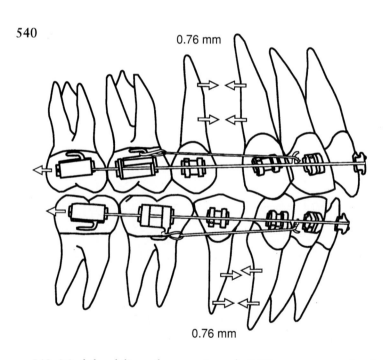

540 Modules delivered approximately 0.76 mm per month of space closure.

541

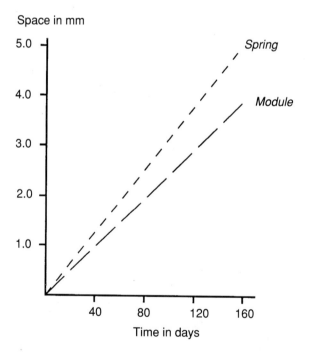

541 Samuels, Rudge and Mair found that springs produced a more rapid rate of space closure.

Samuels, Rudge and Mair also found greater consistency from coil springs (542). They were aware that rapid space closure has been described as producing unwanted effects, due to loss of control of tip and torque and they checked for this.[5] Independent examination was carried out of models and orthopantomograms taken at the time that space closure was achieved, and no clinically detectable difference in tooth positions or angulations could be found. During treatment 'the problems of torque control and excessive gingival tissue accumulating in the extraction sites were not encountered, nor was the tendency towards lateral open bite seen'.

The authors feel that the initial work by Samuels, Rudge and Mair is valuable. It confirms the effectiveness of modules as a method of space closure, and suggests that nickel titanium coils may be even more effective. Clearly, further work will be done in the future to establish even more precisely the optimal force levels and methods of delivering efficient space closure (543). For example, it may be that the more rapid space closure achieved with nickel titanium springs does not allow for adequate torque control of the incisors. This will need to be carefully evaluated.

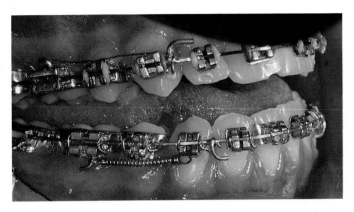

543

543 This case has a passive tieback in place after completion of upper space closure, and a 150 Gm Sentalloy spring for lower space closure.

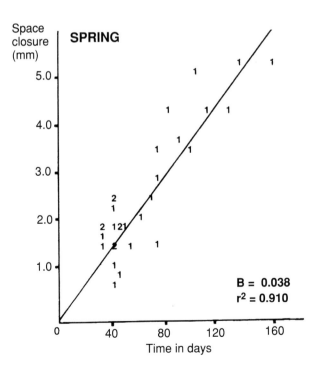

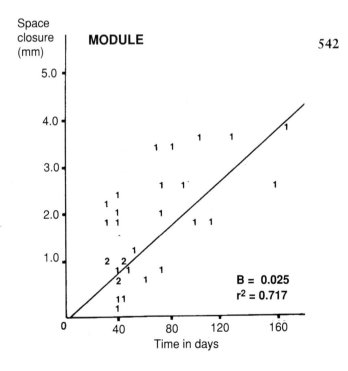

542 Samuels, Rudge and Mair found that springs also showed greater consistency in delivering space closure.

Unwanted Effects of Too Rapid Space Closure

Reduced torque control was noted when space closed more rapidly than 1.5 mm per month. This resulted in upper incisors being too upright at the end of space closure, with spaces distal to canines, and an unesthetic appearance (544). It proved difficult to regain torque which had been lost in this way. Also, rapid mesial movement of upper molars was found to allow palatal cusps to hang down, resulting in functional interferences (545). Rapid movement of lower molars caused rolling. Reduced rotation control during rapid space closure was mainly evident adjacent to extraction sites (546).

544

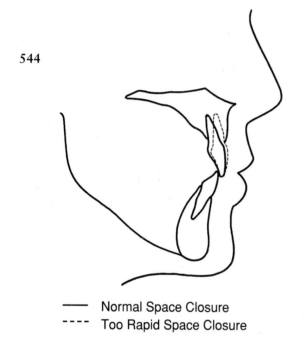

——— Normal Space Closure
- - - - Too Rapid Space Closure

544 Too rapid incisor retraction (---) when compared with normal space closure (—), left incisors with inadequate torque.

545

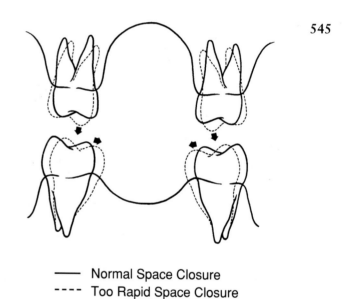

——— Normal Space Closure
- - - - Too Rapid Space Closure

545 Too rapid space closure also allowed unfavorable torque effects on upper and lower molars. The movements shown were not favorable for proper functional chewing movements, and molars in this position required additional torque to reach ideal angulations.

Reduced tip control allowed unwanted effects amongst canines, premolars, and molars, and produced a tendency to lateral open bite. In high angle cases, where lower molars tipped most freely, the elevated distal cusps created the possibility of molar fulcrum effect (547).

Undue soft tissue hyperplasia occurred at the extraction sites during some instances of rapid space closure. As well as being unhygienic, this prevented full space closure, or caused rebound after treatment. In certain cases local gingival surgery was necessary to allow full space closure, or to prevent re-opening.

Appliance variations have been designed to overcome the unwanted consequences of too-rapid tooth movement. These have extra preangulation for tip, rotation and torque. The authors evaluated them. The theoretical benefits were often outweighed by disadvantages during the opening stages of leveling and aligning, when they threatened anchorage more than a standard system. Also, the varied prescriptions required special arrangements for stock control in the office.

Over a 12-year period the authors have independently and together assessed a very wide variety of systems and force levels for achieving space closure. They remain convinced that currently the most efficient method has proved to be sliding mechanics with a standard appliance prescription closing 1.0–1.5 mm of space per month with gentle forces, and paying due regard to possible inhibitors, described overleaf.

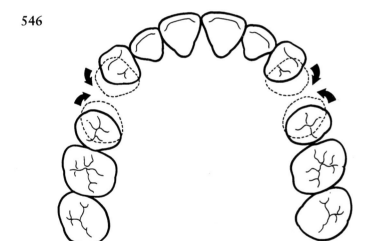

546 In response to too-rapid space closure, it was found that there was an increased tendency for 'rolling in' of teeth adjacent to extraction sites.

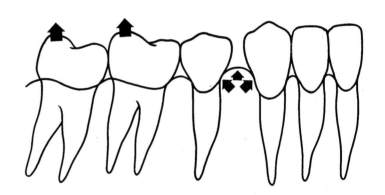

547 Unwanted effects of too rapid space closure included lower molar tipping, with extrusion of the distal cusps, especially in high angle cases. Also, excessive soft tissue build-up occurred, which sometimes prevented proper space closure, or caused re-opening of extraction space.

Overcoming the Possible Inhibitors to Sliding Mechanics

548

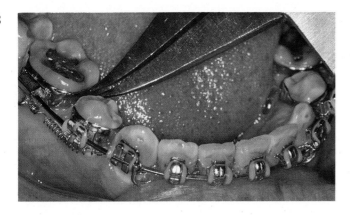

548 It is possible to monitor the rate of space closure by measuring the remaining space. Alternatively, the rectangular wire can be measured as it emerges from the molar tube. This case has a lower second molar bracket on the first molar. This can be helpful in the opening stages of close bite cases, to avoid interferences, before switching bands later in treatment.

In instances where an inhibiting factor appeared to be delaying space closure, it was possible to measure progress in two ways. Calipers were used to directly measure extraction sites, or else the amount of rectangular wire protruding distal to the terminal molar tube was measured at successive visits.

Good alignment of bracket slots was found to be essential for effective sliding mechanics, otherwise residual torque, rotational, or vertical discrepancies produced frictional resistance. The normal procedure was to use .018 round wire for at least one month prior to placement of .019 /.025 rectangular wire. It became clear that levelling and aligning was continuing for at least a month after insertion of rectangular wires and no attempt at space closure was attempted during that time. Newly-placed rectangular wires were tied passively (549), for the first month, and passive ties were continued until all leveling and aligning was felt to be complete, and the rectangular archwires were passively engaged in the brackets and tubes. Conventional elastic tiebacks were then placed (550). In some cases the transition into elastic tiebacks did not take place for three months.

549

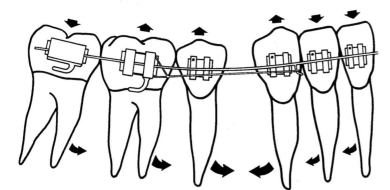

550

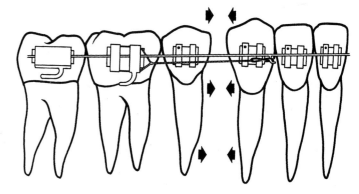

549 Rectangular .019/.025 archwires at the time of placement, with passive tiebacks, awaiting completion of levelling and aligning to achieve passivity of the brackets on the new archwires.

550 Elastic tiebacks in place to commence sliding mechanics in a low friction system, as compared with the high friction system which occurred at the time of placement of rectangular wires.

At the initiation of space closure and throughout this stage of treatment, frictional resistance from three primary sources was possible. These sources were first order or rotational resistance, second order or tipping resistance, and third order or torsional (torque) resistance (**551–3**).

First order or rotational resistance occurred at the mesio-buccal and the disto-lingual aspects of the posterior bracket slots (**551**). The cause of this frictional resistance was related to the application of forces on the buccal aspects of the posterior teeth, creating mesial rotation of these teeth. The most effective method of counteracting this type of frictional resistance was to apply lingual elastic forces intermittently (alternating one month from canine to first molar and the next month from canine to second molar) during space closure.

Second order or tipping resistance occurred at the mesio-occlusal and at the disto-gingival aspects of the posterior bracket slots (**552**). The cause of this frictional resistance was related to excessive forces which caused tipping of the posterior teeth, a lack of rebound time for uprighting of these teeth, and a resultant binding of the system. The importance of applying light forces (of 50–150 Gms) cannot be overemphasized when using this system of mechanics.

Third order or torsional resistance occurred at any one of four areas of the bracket slot where the edges of the rectangular wire made contact (**553**). The cause of this frictional resistance, like that of tipping resistance, was related mainly to excessive forces from overactivated tiebacks. As discussed earlier and illustrated in **545** and **546**, excessive forces caused upper posterior lingual cusps to drop down and lower posterior teeth to roll in lingually.

551   **552**   **553**

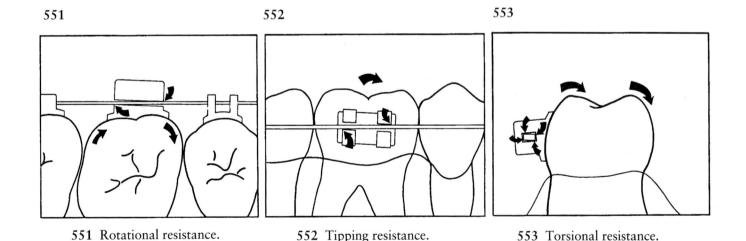

551 Rotational resistance.   552 Tipping resistance.   553 Torsional resistance.

Occasionally a small space would open between the first and second molars during space closure, since forces were directed from first molars to anterior hooks on the archwires. This was managed in one of three ways:

- First and second molars could be laced together before beginning space closure. This technique was also slightly more effective in preserving posterior anchorage.
- A 'K-2' elastic could be extended from the second molar to the hook on the archwire, in addition to the elastic or wire tieback attached to the first molar. This adequately closed the space, but created an additional hygiene concern for the patient.
- The elastic tieback could be extended from the second molar, instead of the first molar, to the hook on the archwire. This was particularly effective after the extraction sites and all other spaces had been closed (554).

Damaged brackets on lower premolars or first molars occasionally caused local hindrance to space closure. Such damage occurred either as a result of careless use of biting sticks during case set-up, or following a lack of dietary care by the patient. Although local thinning of the archwire was found to allow normal space closure to resume, it was generally better to replace the damaged item. Such instances of damage were rare, being seen less than once a month in a typical caseload.

Interference from opposing teeth sometimes restricted lower arch space closure. This occurred particularly if bracket placement was not correct, or if a complete unit Class II relationship existed between upper and lower cheek teeth (555). Correction of band or bracket position normally allowed progress to resume. Occasionally stones were used to selectively remove individual wings of lower brackets. Sometimes one or two lower brackets were removed completely for a few weeks, until the interference was eliminated.

As spaces closed, the ends of the rectangular wires protruded more and more from the distal molar tube. It was found to be helpful for patient comfort to regularly shorten the wires. Also, there was a tendency for protruding wires to be bent gingivally due to chewing forces, if they were allowed to extend more than 2 mm from the distal tube. This prevented easy removal of rectangular wires for adjustment. Anything, such as a ligature wire or an erupting molar, which could restrict the steady emergence of the wire in this way, needed to be identified and eliminated as a potential inhibitor to sliding mechanics.

Generally, it was not found helpful to increase force levels above those provided by a conventional elastic tieback. However, in some low angle adult treatments, levels were increased if lower space closure was not occurring after two months with normal force, applied to fully leveled brackets.

554

555

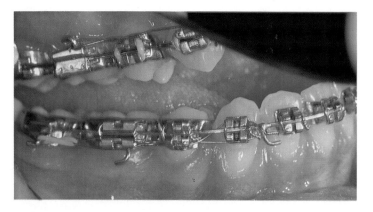

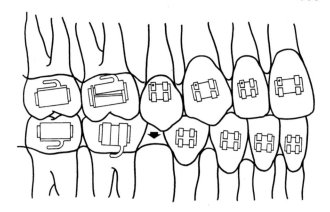

554 In this case the elastic tieback has been extended from the second molar. If the capping is removed from the first molar tube, to convert it to a bracket, it is correct to tie with a wire ligature. An elastomeric module is not strong enough to control the molar tooth.

555 An upper premolar bracket placed too gingivally, preventing lower space closure.

Certain tissue factors at the extraction site sometimes hindered achievement of full space closure, but these did not relate to the particular mechanics used, and might occur with any method of space closure. Soft-tissue build-up as a result of poor plaque control or too-rapid space closure was one factor. Another was a tendency to narrowing of the alveolar cortical plate, mesial to lower first molars, after extraction of second premolars, especially in lower angle situations. Retained roots, ankylosed teeth, and bone sclerosis were among other possible local factors to be considered.

Achieving Anchorage Control

The authors reviewed various methods of anchorage control during space closure. In many cases, after unraveling crowding, there was space available in the extraction sites which could be used to improve denture positioning, and thus enhance the result (556). Where small amounts of space were involved, it was often found unnecessary to alter the reciprocal arrangement. In other instances, proper anchorage control produced a change of balance during space closure, away from the reciprocal closure which could be expected from the arrangement shown in 537 and 538 towards a system which favored distal movement of incisors or molar mesial movement.

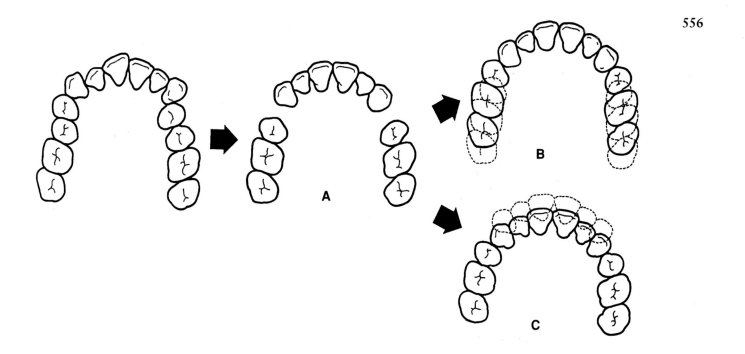

556

556 Anchorage balance possibilities during space closure. In **A** part of the 7 mm space has been used to unravel anterior crowding. Canines have not been moved away from lateral incisors, but have been retracted just enough to allow good alignment of the six front teeth. It was then open to the orthodontist to use anchorage control methods to achieve **B** or **C**, depending on the needs of the case. **B** is normally described as 'anchorage loss' and **C** as 'anchorage gain'.

557

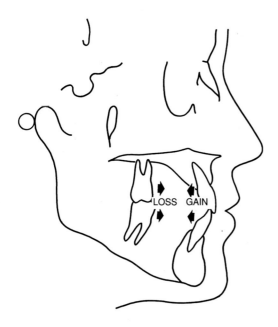

557 Traditional orthodontic terminology has used 'anchorage loss' to describe mesial molar movement, and 'anchorage gain' to describe distal incisor movement. The terms are not entirely logical.

In orthodontic terminology 'anchorage loss' has traditionally been used to describe a situation where molars move forwards in the sagittal plane. 'Anchorage gain' has described backwards movement of incisors (557). The terms are not entirely logical, but will be used in this way in this text. For example 'anchorage loss' in the maxilla is often beneficial in management of Class III problems.

The manœuvres described were normally applicable to maxillary or mandibular treatment mechanics, but where a key difference exists between upper and lower arch mechanics, this has been noted.

In general it was found that there was more anchorage available than might be expected, provided forces were kept light, which has led the authors towards considering the loss of second premolars rather than first premolars in a higher percentage of cases.

Varying the extraction decision gives a convenient and effective method of anchorage control in the maxilla, where loss of first premolars provides more anchorage gain than second premolar extraction. The effect is less clear in the mandible, due to a tendency for the cortical bone to form an 'hourglass' shape, especially in lower angle cases, restricting mesial movement of first molars.

The choice of:

$\frac{5/5}{4/4}$ extractions in Class III cases and

$\frac{4/4}{5/5}$ extractions in Class II division 1 cases

proved generally helpful in balancing anchorage control. Intermaxillary elastics were found to be a convenient and effective method of anchorage control (558). It was found that they could be used routinely at force levels of 100 Gms in average or low angle patterns.

Much more care was needed in higher angle patterns, where the muscular forces were less able to resist the extrusive component of intermaxillary force. In these cases the elastics were used selectively in short spells, sometimes only at night, with force levels reduced to between 50 and 70 Gms.

558

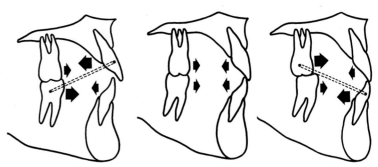

558 Intermaxillary elastics were found to effectively vary anchorage balance, according to the needs of an individual case, during space closure.

Palatal and lingual arches of a rigid, soldered type were found to be effective in supporting anchorage during the opening stages of treatment, when leveling and aligning, and unraveling overcrowding. In general they were not helpful during space closure. Because of group movement of teeth, there was a need to incorporate adjustment loops to avoid frequent impingement of soft or hard tissues, and this reduced their rigidity and effectiveness. The time taken in adjusting palatal and lingual arches during space closure undermined the efficiency of the overall system, and the authors favor other methods of anchorage support at this stage of treatment.

Extra-oral force was found to be effective in controlled space closure. Conventional combination headgear, worn nocturnally, was found to control upper molars via a face bow. The 'J' hook type of headgear was carried directly to archwire hooks in the maxilla in selected cases, with the archwire turned upside-down.

Conventional headgear force was not applied to the mandibular dentition, to avoid the risk of unwanted effects on the temperomandibular joints. Reverse headgears (or face-masks) were well accepted by patients and provided a convenient method of losing or 'burning' anchorage. The elastics were applied either directly to molar hooks, or to archwire hooks after modification. Reverse headgears allowed an asymmetrical force to be provided in some cases where the problem was unilateral or where there was a midline shift.

Lip bumpers were evaluated as a method of anchorage support in the lower arch, and, with good co-operation, supported lower arch anchorage when maximally required. These lip bumpers have actually been used more effectively in non-extraction cases requiring uprighting or distal tipping of lower molars.

Utility arches were occasionally used in the lower arch when incisor intrusion and molar uprighting were indicated. This type of mechanics also provided additional anchorage in the lower arch.

Archwire thinning was evaluated. Although effective, it was discarded in favor of selective torque application, because of the reduced tooth control which resulted in the thinned areas.

Selective torque application to the .019/.025 rectangular wires proved a useful and effective method of anchorage control, especially in the incisor regions (559). It was found that the previously flat wires could be adjusted quickly and easily at the chairside to carry a customized 10–15° of incisor torque. Likewise, molar torque was selectively applied as a measure to resist mesial movement of molars, and create a basis for good functional movements.

559

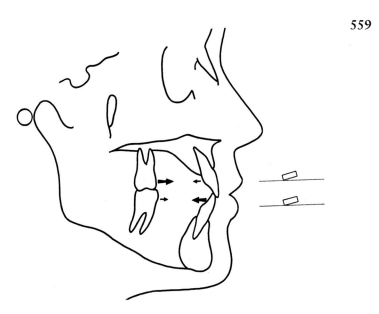

559 When torque was introduced into the rectangular archwires, it affected anchorage balance in both anterior and posterior regions during space closure.

Summary of Key Points

This chapter presents a detailed review of a method of space closure which has proved useful and effective in the authors' hands. The main conclusions may be summarized as follows:

- The details of the recommended mechanics have been shown to be important. Correct archwire size and design, properly designed appliances, and correct force levels are among the factors found to be essential for consistent results. The disadvantages of alternative force delivery systems and of too-rapid space closure have been discussed.
- A list of possible inhibitors to sliding mechanics, and hence proper space closure, has been given. Recommendations have been made, which, if followed, will reduce the likelihoo problems. The key importance of level slot line-up, imp careful leveling and aligning of a well-designed bracke tem, has been stressed.
- Methods of varying anchorage balance have been revie The recommended space closure mechanics are straigh ward and allow the orthodontist time to focus on the in tant aspect of denture positioning. There is scope for fu work to evaluate the effectiveness of various anchorage trol methods, such as the choice of first premolars versu ond premolars in the lower arch, for example.

An edited version of this chapter was first published in 1990, (Bennett, J.C. & McLaughlin R.P., *J. Clin. Orth*. 24: 251–260, 1990) and a fuller version, in German, was published in *Orthodontie und Kieferorthopädie* also in 1990 under the title 'Kontrollierter Lückenschluß mit der Straight-Wire-Apparatur'.

CASE REPORT KL

A Class I low angle case with severe crowding,
treated by the extraction of four first premolars

A girl aged 14 years and 9 months with a Class II skeletal pattern and Class I dental pattern, with severe crowding in the upper and lower anterior regions. Although she was a low angle case, it was necessary to extract four premolars to deal with the crowding.

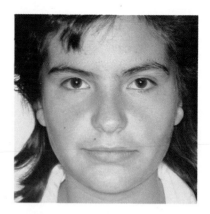

560

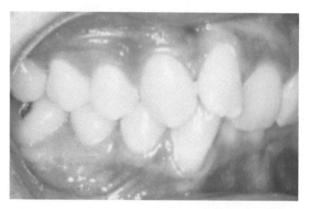

563

Occlusal views confirm the severe anterior crowding. Upper incisors showed typical features of Class II division 2 malocclusion, with retroclined central incisors. There was a high lip line.

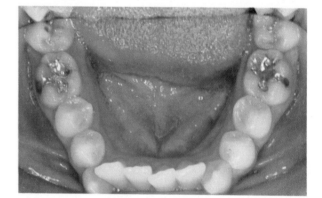

566

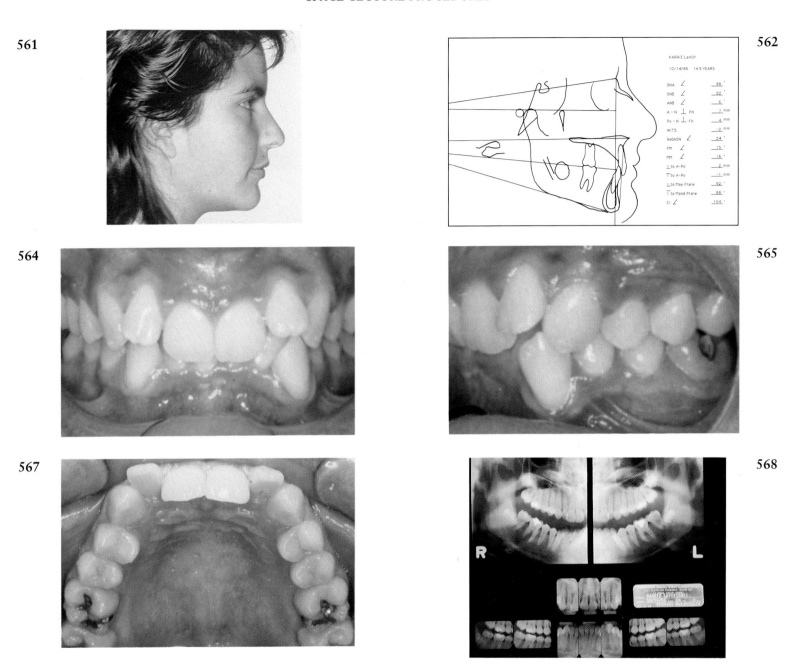

561

562

KARRIE LaVOY

10/14/86 14.9 YEARS

SNA ∠	88 °
SNB ∠	82 °
ANB ∠	6 °
A – N ⊥ FH	7 mm
Po – N ⊥ FH	4 mm
WITS	-2 mm
GoGnSN ∠	24 °
FM ∠	15 °
MM ∠	16 °
1̲ to A-Po	2 mm
1̄ to A-Po	-1 mm
1̲ to Max Plane	92 °
1̄ to Mand Plane	88 °
CI ∠	104 °

564

565

567

568

R L

Lacebacks were used, with light initial forces. Both upper lateral incisors were bracketed, and modules were placed to protect the soft tissues. Bracketing of these teeth could have been delayed for two or three months.

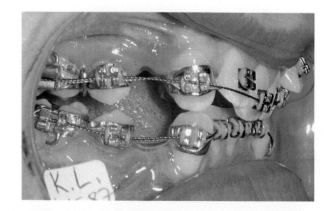

569

A removable acrylic bite plate was used for early control of the overbite.

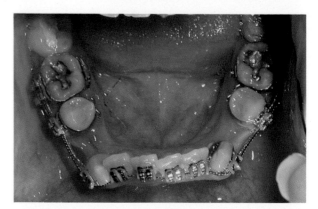

572

After three and a half months of treatment, light round wires were fully engaged into the brackets. Lacebacks were still in place at this stage.

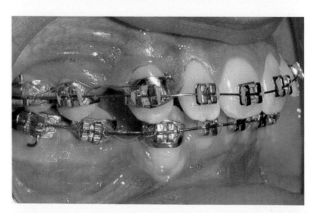

575

After five months of treatment a lower rectangular .019/.025 wire was placed, with passive tiebacks. The upper wire is .018 round.

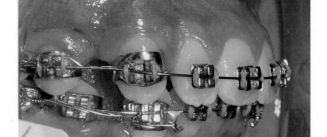

578

570

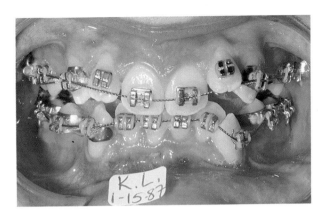

571

573

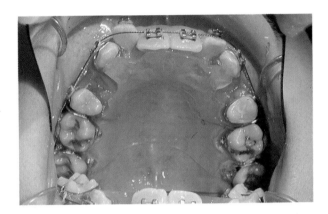

574

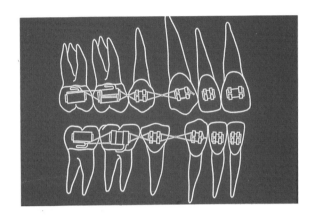

576

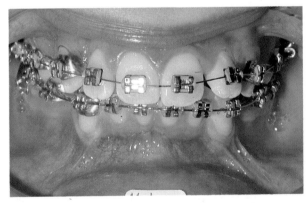

577

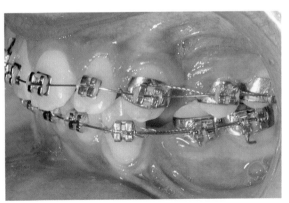

579

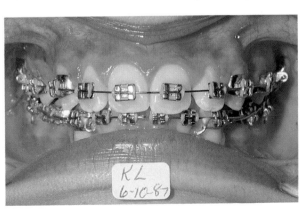

580

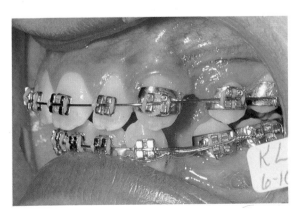

Space closure was carried out with .019/.025 rectangular wires and elastic tiebacks, as described in Chapter 10. Torque control was maintained by adding labial root torque in the lower incisor region, and palatal root torque in the upper incisor region.

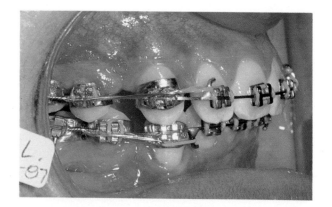

581

The patient wore light Class II elastics, and the archwires were adjusted to control the curve of Spee. Elastic tiebacks were slightly tighter than normal during space closure in this low angle case. Care was taken to avoid unwanted effects (587).

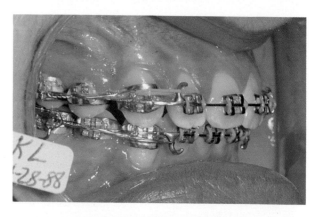

584

Upper and lower rectangular wires are shown in 588. There is exaggerated curve of Spee in the upper wire, and torque has been left without adjustment anteriorly. There is anti-Spee curvature in the lower, and torque needs to be adjusted to zero in the incisor region before placement. Wires are flat for the first one or two months, and after that 2 or 3 mm of curvature may be added to assist overbite control.

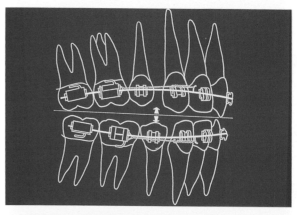

587

Lower space closure has been completed, and passive tiebacks are in place. Active upper tiebacks are being used to complete upper space closure.

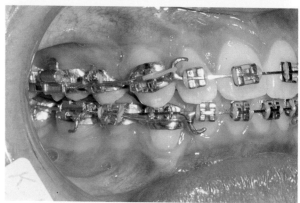

590

582
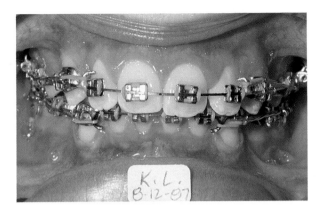

583
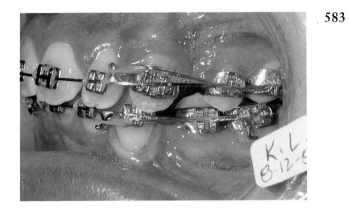

585
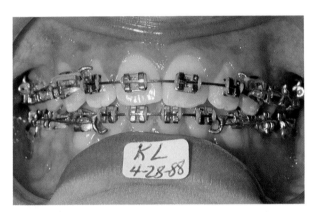

586
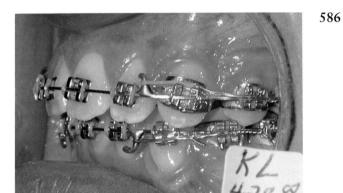

588
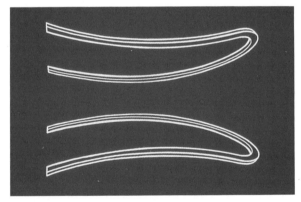

589
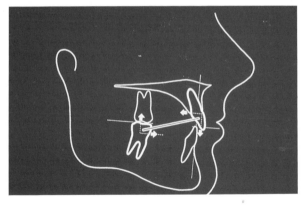

591
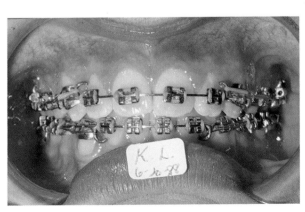

592
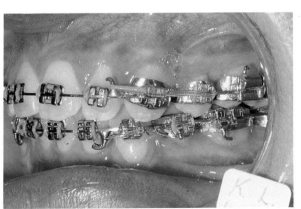

Final space closure was carried out slowly and carefully to preserve facial profile and control the overbite.

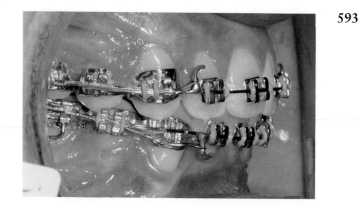

593

A lower premolar-to-premolar retainer was cemented in place. The patient was asked to wear a nocturnal removable upper Hawley retainer.

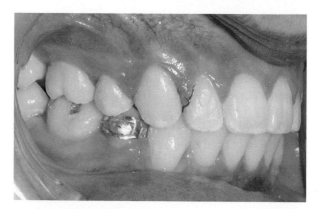

596

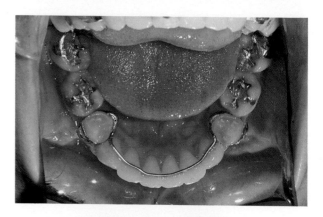

599

Final X-rays show that good vertical control was maintained in this low angle extraction case.

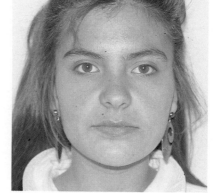

601

594

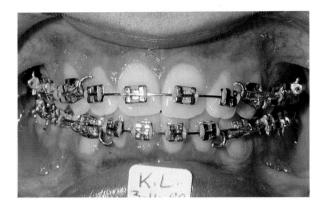

595

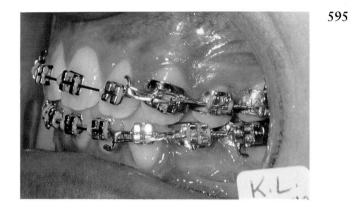

597

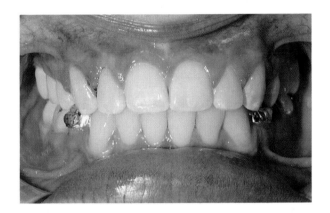

598

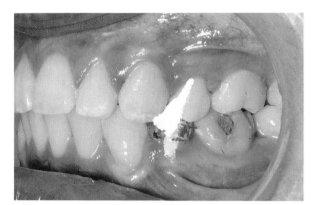

600

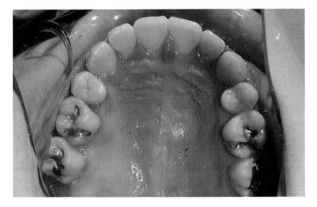

602

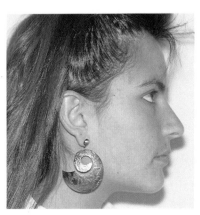

603

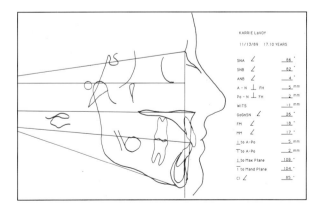

KARRIE LaVOY

11/13/89   17.10 YEARS

SNA ∠	86 °
SNB ∠	82 °
ANB ∠	4 °
A - N ⊥ FH	5 mm
Po - N ⊥ FH	2 mm
WITS	-1 mm
GoGnSN ∠	26 °
FM ∠	18 °
MM ∠	17 °
⊥ to A-Po	5 mm
⊤ to A-Po	2 mm
⊥ to Max Plane	108 °
⊤ to Mand Plane	104 °
CI ∠	85 °

11. FINISHING AND DETAILING

Introduction

In previous chapters the authors have described the management of various stages of orthodontic treatment using the preadjusted appliance system. An attempt was made to objectively point out the advantages and disadvantages of such appliance systems, but it is widely accepted that preadjusted appliances have provided great benefits to the orthodontic profession in all stages of treatment.

Theoretically, however, these appliances should provide their greatest benefit in the finishing and detailing stages of treatment. If the tip, torque and in-out compensation built into the appliance is accurately suited to the patient's dentition, and the brackets are properly positioned, as treatment proceeds towards completion, there should be only minimal wire bending required to complete the treatment.

The actual amount of finishing and detailing required at the end of treatment with the preadjusted appliance may be increased by any of the following variables:

- Variations in the shape and size of the patient's teeth relative to the average measurements built into the preadjusted appliance.

- Inaccuracies or shortcomings in appliance design. As a result the three-dimensional forces delivered by the appliance do not produce accurate tooth positioning.
- Use of force levels that 'overpower' the selected appliance design.
- Inaccuracies in appliance placement.
- Failure to allow sufficient time for the bracket system to express itself. (Leaving the appliance in place for a further three months after main corrections are complete, and re-tying at monthly intervals, will often allow time for the brackets to produce additional favorable tooth movements.)

In 1976, Dougherty described 17 factors that should be considered in the finishing and detailing stage of orthodontic treatment.[1] The purpose of this chapter will be to review these factors as they relate to the preadjusted appliance system and the above five variables.

Correction and Overcorrection of the Antero-Posterior Jaw Relationship

Most of these comments are not specific to preadjusted appliance systems. The tip and torque built into the anterior brackets place a greater initial demand on anchorage, particularly in the upper arch. However, the *total* anchorage required to correct antero-posterior jaw relationship is the same with all appliances, if teeth are moved from the initial irregularity to the same fully corrected final position.

The need for overcorrection of the Class II case is the greatest orthodontic challenge in this area.

Many Class II cases, if only corrected to the desired end-position, will show relapse, with the overjet returning and usually the bite deepening. These patients benefit from over-correction to an end-to-end position, and maintenance of that position with night time Class II elastics for six to eight weeks, which is followed by settling into an ideal Class I relationship.

Other corrected Class II cases occasionally show a Class III growth tendency in retention and clearly do not benefit from overcorrection in the finishing stage of treatment.

This entire area of growth prediction is a difficult one and, as mentioned above, is unrelated to any particular appliance system.

Establishing Correct Tip of the Upper and Lower Anterior Teeth

The introduction of tip into the face of preadjusted appliance brackets has allowed for correction of tip in the upper and lower anterior segments with very little effort. This tip built into the face of the brackets has eliminated the need for second order or 'beauty' bends in the anterior segments and therefore allows for much greater efficiency in treatment. Wire bending to establish proper anterior tip is required in only two specific situations:

- When brackets are improperly placed relative to the vertical reference lines of the anterior teeth. (It is much easier to reposition brackets rather than placing unnecessary bends in the anterior segments of the upper and lower archwires.)

- Irregularly shaped anterior teeth. (There are instances where second order anterior bends are required to compensate for irregularly shaped anterior teeth such as peg shaped lateral incisors.)

When there is anterior spacing, there is also a mechanical advantage to having tip built into anterior brackets. Because there are no anterior archwire bends, the brackets slide along the wire more efficiently. This 'straight' archwire therefore allows sliding mechanics when needed for closure of anterior space.

Establishing Correct Torque of the Upper and Lower Anterior Teeth

The upper and lower anterior torque needs of patients vary greatly, so that there is no single torque value that can be recommended for upper and lower incisor brackets for the large variety of cases seen in an orthodontic practice. Therefore, it is often necessary to adjust the torque in the rectangular archwires in the upper and lower anterior segments at various stages of treatment. This is likely to be necessary in treatment of a moderate to severe Class II problem (604), in which torque is frequently lost in the upper anteri-

or segment during overjet correction, with the lower incisors becoming angulated forward during the same correction (605). In this situation it is often necessary to add lingual root torque to the upper anterior archwire and labial root torque to the lower anterior archwire (606). This compensation should be placed in the archwires early in space closure and overjet correction rather than attempting to re-establish proper torque that has been lost.

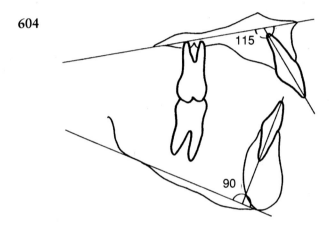

604 Start malocclusion.

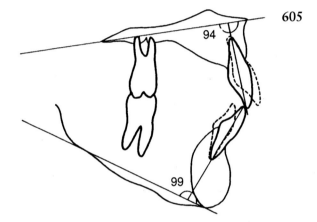

605 Teeth at the end of overjet reduction in which torque has been lost in the upper anterior segment and the lower incisors are angulated forward.

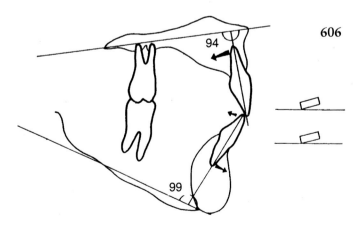

606 Torque which needs to be added to the archwires to attempt to recover correct incisor angulation. This wire bending ideally should be carried out in the very early stages of space closure and overjet reduction.

Co-ordinating Arch Widths and Form

Upper and lower archwires should be co-ordinated from the early stages of treatment through to the rectangular wire stage. This will help eliminate unwanted and troublesome crossbites in the finishing stages. Most arch width discrepancies can be fully corrected by the time the rectangular wire stage has been reached. This can be achieved by noting any lack of co-ordination in the patient's arch width at the beginning of treatment, and by narrowing or widening the appropriate archwires from the outset. With some asymmetry cases, the patient's archform may show distortion in the anterior segments, particularly in the canine areas. This can be treated by using cross elastics in the canine areas (**607**) and by canting the archwires in the opposite direction to the arch asymmetry (**608**). Archwire canting and elastic wear will often help correction of anterior asymmetries even before the finishing stages of treatment.

607

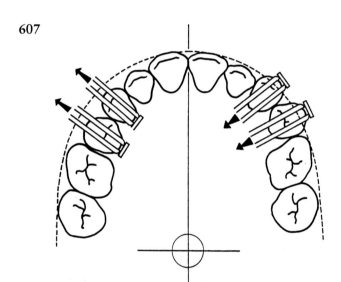

607 An asymmetrical upper arch compared with a symmetrical line (- - - - - -). Cross elastics may be used as shown to enhance the correction.

608

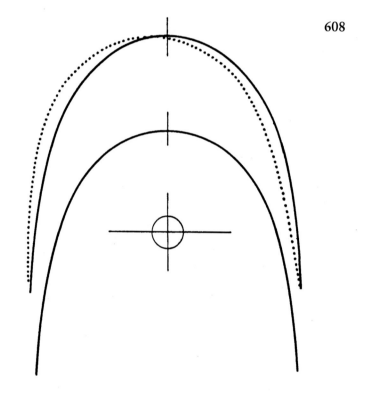

608 Modified upper archform (·····) which may be used to compensate for the type of asymmetry in **607**

Establishing Correct Posterior Crown Torque

Correct posterior crown torque is essential in preventing posterior interferences and allowing for the seating of centric cusps. The torque built into posterior brackets eliminates the need for archwire bends in most situations. However, there is often a tendency for upper palatal cusps to be below the occlusal plane so that posterior buccal root torque needs to be added to the rectangular wires in the finishing stages (609). In the lower arch, first and second molars can show undesirable lingual tipping and it may be necessary to add buccal crown torque to the rectangular archwires in the lower molar regions.

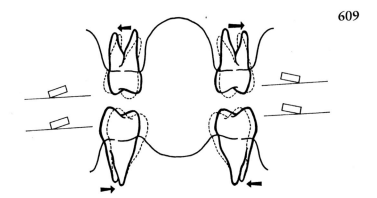

609 Type of torque which needs to be applied to adjust molar root torque during the finishing stages.

Establishing Marginal Ridge Relationships and Contact Points

Marginal ridge relationships are mainly determined by bracket heights during the finishing stage of treatment. The most common method of measuring bracket heights with the standard edgewise appliance involved measuring a specific distance from the incisor or occlusal surface of each tooth. For example, upper central incisor brackets were frequently placed 5 mm above the incisal edge of the tooth. When the patient's teeth were large, the bracket was placed more incisally when compared to a patient with small teeth (610).

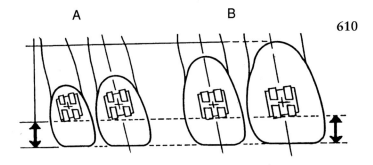

610 Brackets at 5 mm on 8 mm central incisors (A), compared with (B) where brackets at 5 mm are placed on 12 mm central incisors. In A the brackets are 62% up the crown surface compared with 42% in B. These positions introduce possible torque and marginal ridge errors compared with a consistent 50% position originally recommended by Andrews.

This variation in relative position on the teeth from patient to patient resulted in variations in the in/out position of the brackets, and in the amount of torque provided by them, because they were positioned at different thicknesses and curvatures on the teeth. Compensation for these variations was provided as part of the first, second, and third order archwire bending which was routinely needed for standard edgewise treatment.

However, when an attempt was made to design a pre-angulated appliance system that minimized archwire bending for the greatest possible number of patients, a better system of bracket placement was needed. A more reliable and logical position was the center of the clinical crowns, as described by Andrews[2] which provided a similar bracket position in patients with large or small teeth (611). Hence this position was accepted as the horizontal reference plane for preadjusted brackets.

If bracket height is not correct, it becomes apparent during the early stages of leveling and aligning. It is better to reposition these brackets at this early stage of treatment, so that time is not wasted stepping archwires or repositioning brackets during the finishing stages of treatment. The authors have found it helpful to use the .014 round wire to step any brackets that are not properly positioned in terms of horizontal height. At the subsequent visit these brackets can be repositioned with very little loss in treatment time (612 and 613).

There are other times during treatment when brackets can be repositioned, to save time during finishing and detailing. For example, when previously unerupted teeth are bracketed, it is normally necessary to return to a smaller archwire, and any incorrectly placed brackets can be re-positioned at the same appointment. An example would be when second molars erupt enough to allow banding.

611

612

613

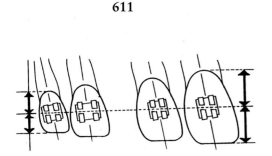 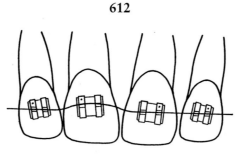 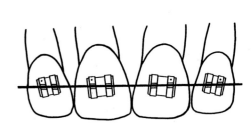

611 is to be compared with **610** and shows recommended 50% positioning in the centers of the clinical crowns, to give consistent torque and marginal ridge factors.

612 Incorrect positioning of an upper central incisor bracket, with a compensating step in the .014 archwire.

613 Bracket subsequently repositioned and a new, heavier archwire in place, with no loss of treatment time.

Correction of Midline Discrepancies

Most minor midline discrepancies of 3 mm or less can be easily corrected in the finishing stages of treatment. Figures **614–618**, on this and the following page, show five methods of elastic wear to correct minor midline discrepancies at the rectangular wire stage:

- A single Class II elastic on one side and a double Class II elastic on the other in cases that have a Class II component (**614**).
- A single Class II elastic on one side when the other side is Class I, and the overjet results from a slight Class II position on one side only (**615**).
- Class III elastics on one side and Class II elastics on the opposing side, when the patient has a Class II dental relationship on one side and a Class III dental relationship on the opposing side (**616**).

- A Class III elastic on one side when that side is Class III, and the opposing side is in a Class I dental relationship (**617**).
- An anterior cross elastic when the discrepancy occurs primarily in the anterior segments rather than the posterior segments (**618**). Asymmetrical elastics should be used for a minimal amount of time, and only with rectangular wires, because of the tendency to cant the occlusal plane. The archwires should be tied back while asymmetrical elastics are worn, so that they do not slide around the arch, causing unwanted space opening and distortion of the archform.

The discussion of midline discrepancies of more than 3 mm is beyond the scope of this chapter, because they require attention before the finishing stages of treatment.

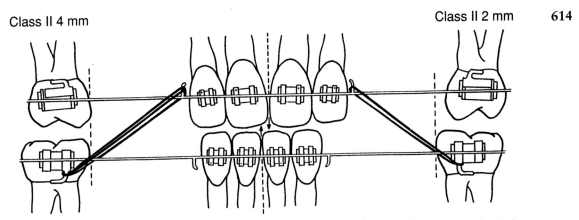

614 A case with a Class II component bilaterally, with a double Class II elastic on the right side and single Class II elastic on the left side.

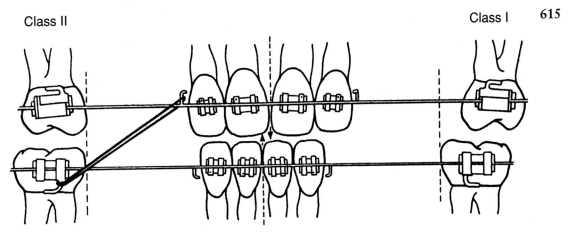

615 A case with Class II molar relationship on the right side and Class I molar relationship on the left side. One Class II elastic is employed on the right side.

616   Class II   Class III

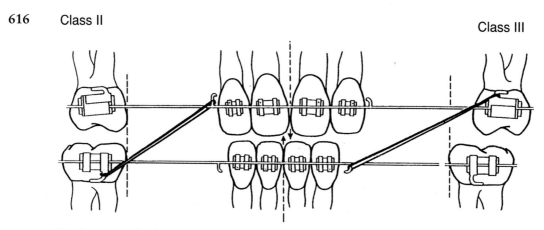

616 A case with class II molar relationship on the right and Class III molar relationship on the left side. Appropriate intermaxillary elastics are used.

617   Class I   Class III

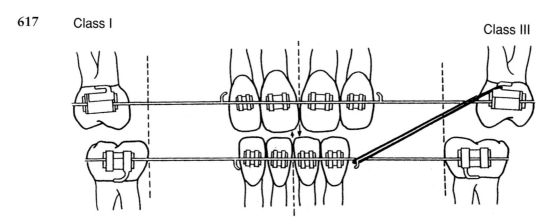

617 A case with Class I dental relationship on the right side and Class III molar relationship on the left side. A single Class III elastic is used on the left.

618   Class I   Class I

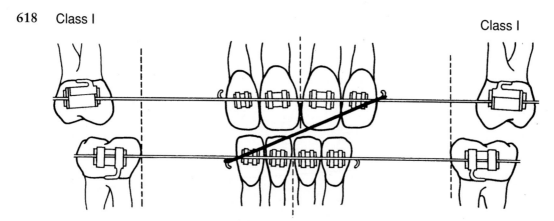

618 An anterior cross elastic in a case where the discrepancy is in the anterior segments, rather than the posterior segments. This should be used only with rectangular wires, and for a minimal amount of time, to avoid cant of the occlusal plane. Tiebacks have not been shown in **614–618** to assist clarity of the drawings but they are needed in all the examples to prevent archwires sliding around.

Establishing the Interdigitation of Teeth

Frequently when rectangular wires have been in position for a long time, teeth are unable to properly settle into an ideal finishing position. Therefore, the authors allow each case to settle prior to debanding in the finishing stages of treatment using a .014 round wire in the lower arch and a .014 upper sectional wire from lateral incisor to lateral incisor.[3] This is accompanied by the use of vertical triangular elastics (**619**), which encourage the teeth to individually settle into position prior to debanding. Once this settling procedure has been allowed to work for 2–4 weeks, then the occlusion can be re-evaluated. If the teeth have settled properly into position, the patient can be scheduled for debanding. If they are not

properly positioned, then the patient can return to heavier archwires for finishing procedures. It may also be necessary in this situation to reposition brackets, but this should normally be done at an earlier stage of treatment. If cases settle without having rectangular wires in position, they are allowed to establish their own individualized archform, within certain limits.

The archform used during treatment may be slightly wider or narrower than the patient's starting archform. The settling phase allows for correction of minor variations, and retainers will fit better than they would if the patient had moved from rectangular wires directly into retention.

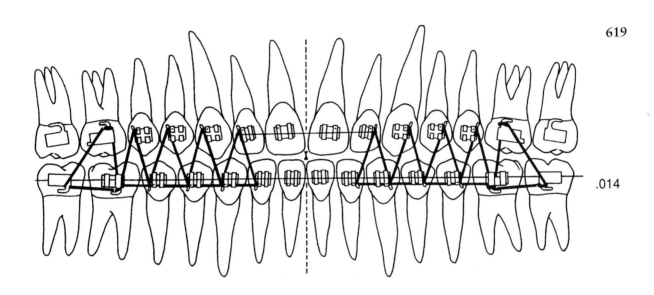

619

.014

619 Vertical triangular elastics in place. Kobyashi hooks are not essential if there is no archwire in place, as vertical elastics may be easily attached to bracket wings (see **632–634**).

215

Checking Cephalometric Objectives

It is often helpful to take progress headfilms approximately halfway through orthodontic treatment to determine how the skeletal and dental component of the patient's problem is being managed. Progress headfilms allow for reassessment of anchorage factors and help revisions in treatment planning as treatment proceeds. The authors also often take final cephalometric headfilms approximately 3–4 months *before debanding,* rather than after treatment. Taking headfilms at the completion of treatment is beneficial from a learning standpoint for future cases, as well as to evaluate the success or failure of the treatment, but it *provides no specific advantage for the patient.* It is better to take the headfilm before debanding so that tooth positions can be corrected before the appliances are removed.

The most important factors to be evaluated with these progress and final cephalometric X-rays involve the antero-posterior position of the incisors, the angulation of the incisors, the changes in the occlusal plane of the patient, the degree to which vertical development of the patient has occurred or been restricted, and the success in correcting the horizontal skeletal and dental component of the patient's problem. It is best to superimpose progress and final X-rays with the initial cephalometric X-ray to accurately determine the changes that have occurred orthodontically.

Checking the Parallelism of Roots

With preadjusted appliance systems, the tip built into the brackets normally provides for proper parallelism of roots. One of the great challenges with the standard edgewise appliances was to properly upright and parallel roots in extraction sites. This has become much less of a problem with the preadjusted appliance system and in fact, in the upper arch particularly, the cuspid can be overtipped to the point where it makes contact with the bicuspid roots.

A panorex X-ray taken prior to debanding is beneficial for evaluation of the parallelism of roots. There are situations where angulation between the crowns and the roots of teeth vary beyond the standard or the norm. When this does occur there may be the need for bracket repositioning or archwire bending to modify these root positions.

Maintaining the Closure of All Spaces

It is most important, particularly in extraction cases, that space closure be maintained with tiebacks during the finishing stages of treatment (620). These passive wire tiebacks are very effective. If this is not done, spaces frequently open in the finishing stages of treatment and need to be re-closed. Also, in extraction cases when there is reason to drop to a smaller archwire for re-leveling procedures or picking up teeth that were previously unerupted, it is beneficial to use lacebacks from molars to cuspids until the rectangular wire stage is resumed (621). The use of lacebacks with light archwires, and passive wire tiebacks with rectangular wires, eliminates this troublesome problem of spaces opening in the finishing stages of treatment.

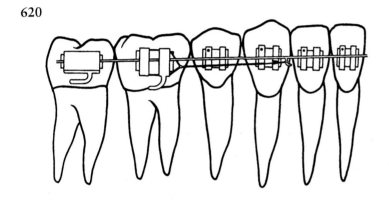

620

620 Lower arch space closure being maintained by the use of a passive tieback between the molar bracket and the soldered archwire hook.

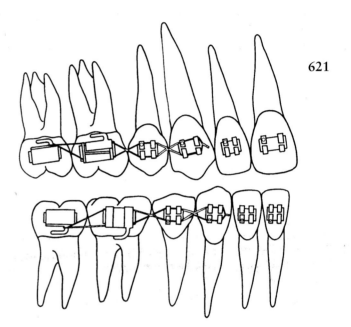

621

621 Lacebacks placed in upper and lower arches maintain space closure when dropping into smaller archwires during finishing procedures.

Evaluating Facial and Profile Esthetics

Evaluation of facial and profile esthetics is an ongoing process during all stages of orthodontic treatment. It is initially evaluated and a projection is made concerning the desired goal of treatment. This esthetic goal can be monitored clinically, as well as with progress and final cephalometric X-rays.

Checking for Temporomandibular Joint Dysfunction, such as Clicking and Locking

This is a large subject that requires more discussion than is possible in this chapter. However, in general, it is most beneficial to:

- Document any evidence of TMJ dysfunction *prior to treatment* and inform the patient that such symptoms do exist.
- Monitor each patient during treatment to determine if any temporomandibular joint symptoms do occur. If these developing problems are managed when they first occur prior to the formation of true internal derangement, then frequently a normal temporomandibular joint function can be re-established without permanent damage. This treatment most commonly involves a short phase of splint therapy during orthodontic treatment in conjunction with physical therapy until the symptoms have been eliminated. Then orthodontic treatment can proceed in a normal fashion with most patients. It is also beneficial if symptoms do occur to eliminate the use of all forces, such as headgear and elastics while resolving the TMJ problem.
- Monitor the patients during the retention phase of treatment to determine if TMJ symptoms occur. The use of tomographic X-rays prior to orthodontic treatment, as well as 3–4 months prior to debanding is helpful in evaluating the presence of irregularities within the structure of the joint and also to evaluate the patient's clinical condyle position.

It is generally accepted that a seated and reasonably concentric condyle position is the most beneficial position to establish during orthodontic treatment. Thus, if the patient shows a forward or retruded condyle position, this can be related to the clinical evaluation of the patient's antero-posterior and vertical jaw positions. In most cases minor changes can be made during the finishing stage of teatment to allow for correction. For example, if the patient shows an anterior skid with a corresponding anterior condyle position, it is beneficial to continue with headgear or Class II mechanics for an additional period of time to eliminate the anterior skid and allow the condyle to seat in the fossa (**622a**). Conversely, if the patient shows a significantly posterior condylar position with no evidence of an anterior skid whatsoever, it is beneficial to provide a slight amount of anterior skid so that the condyle can be in a more centered position. This may be achieved by ceasing Class II elastics or headgear, or by the use of Class III elastics, and is particularly important in cases that show a Class III growth tendency (**622b**).

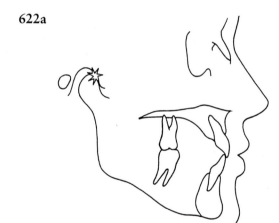

622a If the patient shows an anterior skid with a corresponding anterior condyle position, it is beneficial to continue with headgear or Class II mechanics for an additional period of time to eliminate the anterior skid and allow the condyle to seat in the fossa.

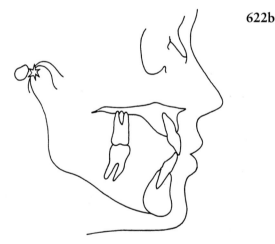

622b If the patient shows a significantly posterior condylar position with no evidence of an anterior skid whatsoever, it is beneficial to provide a slight amount of anterior skid so that the condyle can be in a more centered position. This may be achieved by ceasing Class II elastics or headgear, or by the use of Class III elastics, and is particularly important in cases that show a developing Class III tendency.

Finally, if the condyle is in a reasonably concentric position, with no clinical evidence of an anterior skid, the patient can be debanded and left in that position. This should allow normal TMJ development and function after orthodontic treatment. While we cannot predict the physical and emotional stress levels that will occur with our patient, we can provide the most satisfactory structural environment to best withstand these stressful forces.

Checking Functional Movements

Before debanding, the patient should be checked for interferences during protrusive movements and lateral excursions. During protrusive movements, it is important that the lower eight most anterior teeth make contact with the upper six most anterior teeth as described by Roth.[4] This normally requires slight widening of the archform in the bicuspid area in order that the mesial of the lower bicuspids make contact with the distal of the upper cuspids. During lateral excursions, the patient should experience cuspid rise with slight anterior contact and disclusion of posterior teeth on both the working and balancing sides. Preadjusted orthodontic appliances are most helpful in these areas since they do provide for anterior torque adjustment, as well as posterior torque adjustment, which is critical in the establishing of an ideal functional occlusion.

It is important that second molars normally be banded and correctly positioned to prevent interferences in this critical area during lateral excursions.

Correction of Habits

Various habits, such as tongue thrusting, have normally been corrected prior to the finishing stages of treatment. This is due to two main factors:

- As the patient grows, the airway size is increased and the tongue is allowed to assume a more posterior position.

- As the dental environment is improved orthodontically, the tongue and lip musculature have the opportunity to adapt to this improved environment, and normal function can begin to occur.

The authors have observed that approximately 80% of tongue thrusting habits will self-correct prior to the finishing stages of treatment. Those that tend to persist can be referred for myofunctional therapy during the finishing stages of treatment. Occasionally, if a severe tongue thrusting habit is present, these patients can be referred for myofunctional therapy in the initial stages of treatment, or even before orthodontic treatment.

CASE REPORT IH

A non-extraction case to show the use of
vertical triangular elastics for settling
during finishing and detailing

A boy aged 11.9 years with a Class II molar relationship. The case was managed on a non-extraction basis.

623

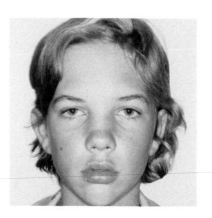

Overbite is slightly deep, with a midline discrepancy of 2 mm.

626

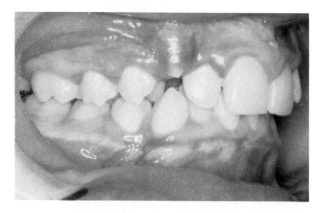

Mirror views from the occlusal show mild upper and lower anterior crowding, with a lack of space for upper canines.

629

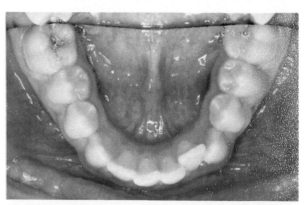

Light round archwires and elastics in place, after 22 months of treatment. The upper sectional wire controls incisor rotations.

632

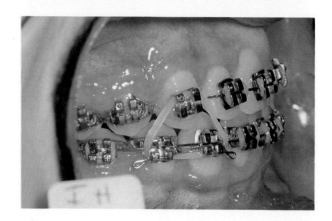

624

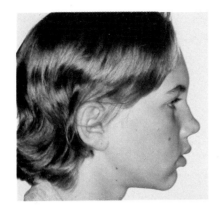

625

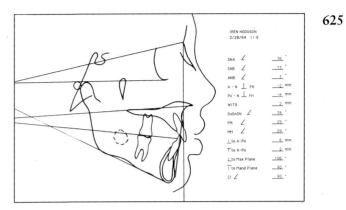

627

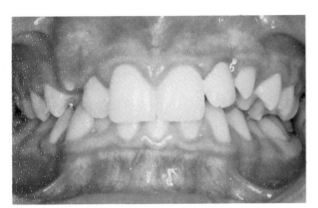

628

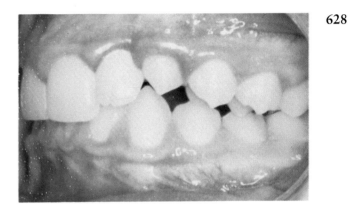

630

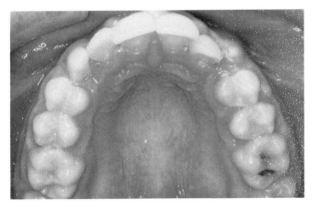

631

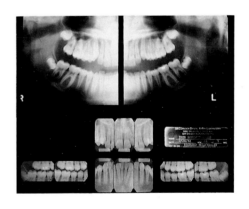

633

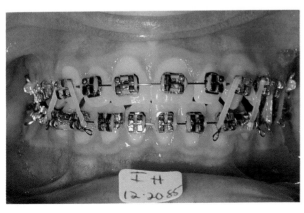

634

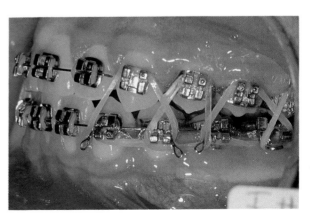

After 22.5 months. There has been settling for approximately ten days. The authors recommend a very light flexible wire for the lower arch such as an .014 nickel titanium wire or an .014 stainless steel wire and a 2 x 2 sectional wire in the upper anterior segment. The buccal segments are treated using light triangular elastics. These elastics are used for only about 7–10 days full time. Once the case is settled, then elastics are worn at night-time for another 7–10 days and then deband procedures can be carried out.

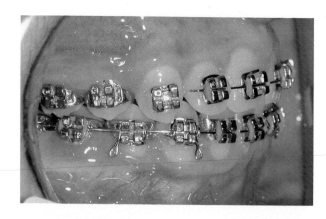

635

The increased overbite and anterior crowding was successfully resolved, and the midline was fully corrected.

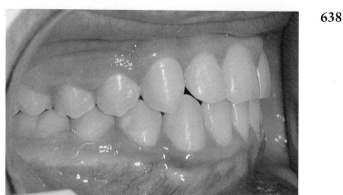

638

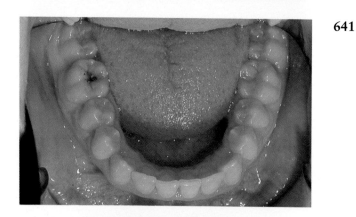

641

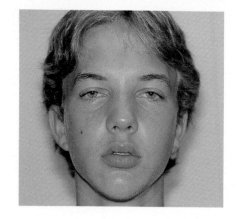

644

636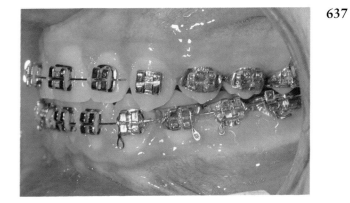

637

639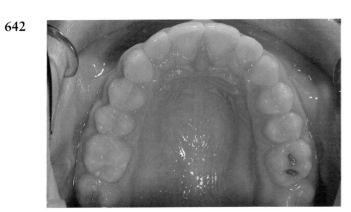

640

642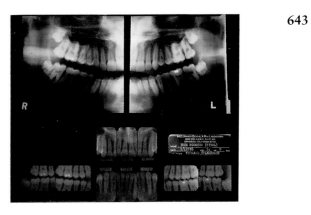

643

645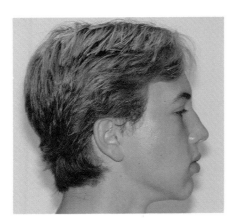

646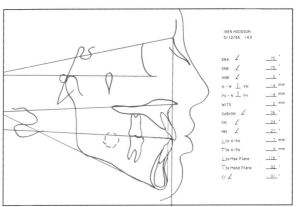

CASE REPORT BS

A case to show anterior torque needs
during the later stages of treatment

A girl aged 11 years and 7 months with a Class II division 1 malocclusion.

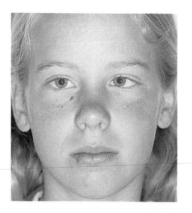

647

She showed an average MM angle with crowding in the upper and lower anterior segments, and as a result, it was decided to extract four first premolars.

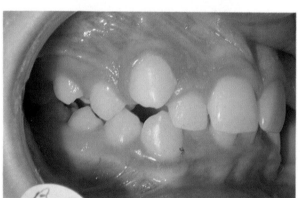

650

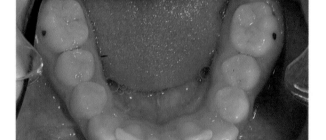

653

648

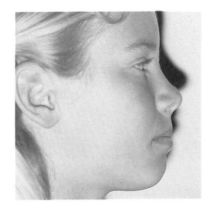

649

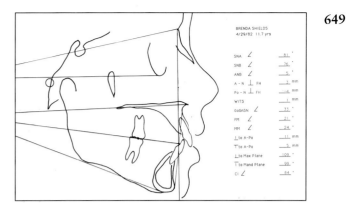

651

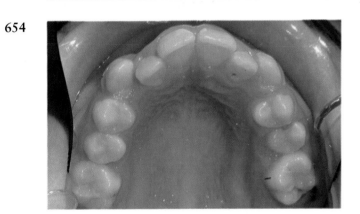

652

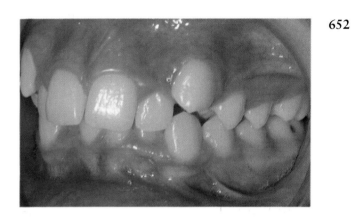

654

After 14 months of treatment, spaces were closed and rectangular wires were in place. However, incisor torque was not correct. Upper palatal root torque and lower buccal root torque was needed. This case was treated in the early 1980s, using incisor brackets with specifications the same as the non-orthodontic normals. Also, at that time, the authors were continuing to evaluate power arms, but they have since stopped using them for reasons discussed in Chapter 2.

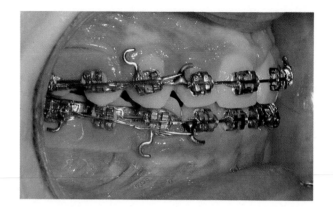

655

Torque was bent into the incisor region of upper and lower archwires. Bends of this type are needed much less frequently if incisor brackets are used with the torque prescription recommended in Chapter 3.

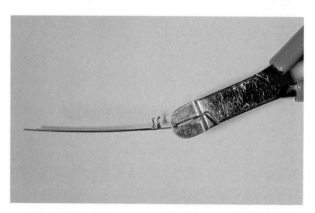

658

Six months later the incisor torque has been corrected, allowing achievement of a proper buccal occlusion.

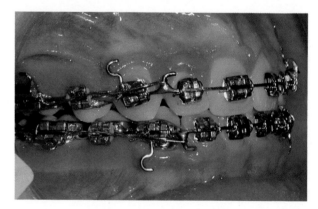

661

656

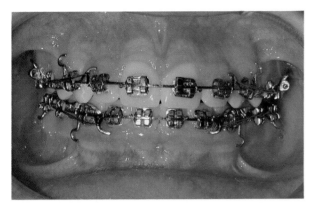

657

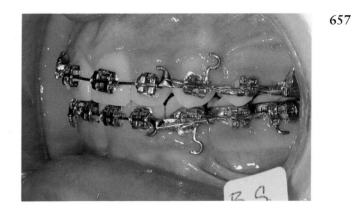

659

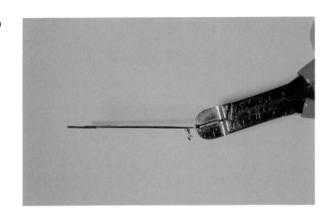

660

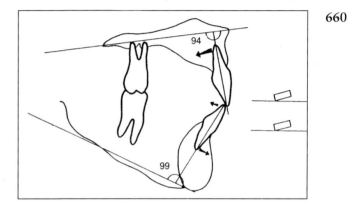

662

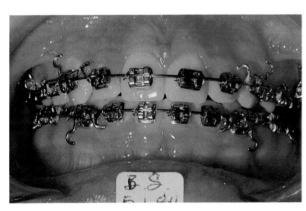

663

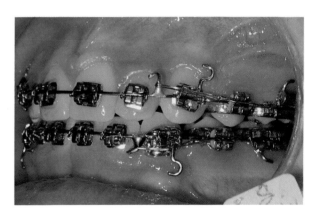

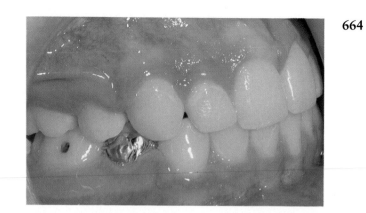

An upper removable Hawley retainer was worn at night. A fixed lower premolar-to-premolar retainer was placed.

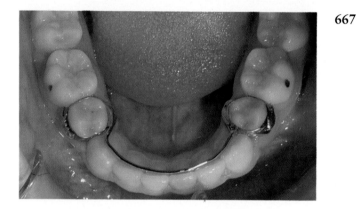

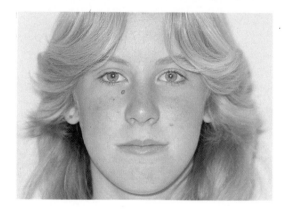

665

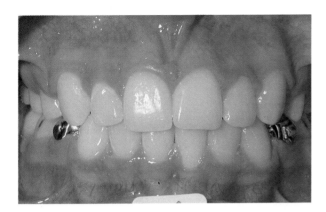

666

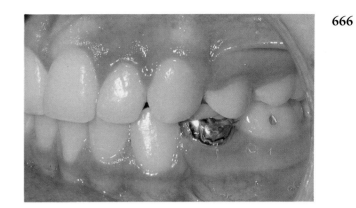

668

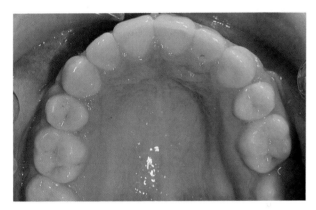

670

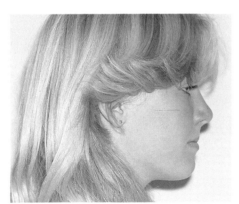

671

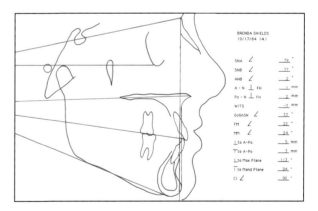

BRENDA SHIELDS
10/17/84 14.1

SNA ∠	79	°
SNB ∠	77	°
ANB ∠	2	°
A - N ⊥ FH	1	mm
Po - N ⊥ FH	2	mm
WITS	-3	mm
GoGnSN ∠	33	°
FM ∠	22	°
MM ∠	24	°
1 to A-Po	5	mm
1 to A-Po	3	mm
1 to Max Plane	113	°
1 to Mand Plane	94	°
CI ∠	90	°

12. NON-EXTRACTION TREATMENT

Introduction

The previous chapters of this text have described mechanical procedures involved in the management of the preadjusted appliance system. The transition from the standard edgewise appliance to preadjusted appliance systems was first discussed and then followed by a review of the six stages of orthodontic treatment as it applies to both extraction and non-extraction cases. There has been, however, an emphasis on extraction treatment, because the mechanics are more complicated than those of non-extraction treatment.

Because of this, the impression may have been given that the authors lean towards extraction treatment and treat an above average number of cases with the extraction of teeth. This is not so, and every attempt is made to treat as many cases as possible on a non-extraction basis. If an unsatisfactory end-result can be anticipated following non-extraction treatment, then extractions are carried out. Although the authors have made no specific analysis of their practices, it is estimated that 70–80% of cases are treated on a non-extrac-

tion basis. Thus, in the last chapter of this text, specific comments are made concerning non-extraction treatment.

In general, when cases present with average to low mandibular plane angles, every attempt is made to treat on a non-extraction basis (672). However, when low angle cases show excessive protrusion and/or crowding, extraction treatment must be carried out. In such cases, care must be taken to avoid vertical collapse following extraction of premolars, and the mechanics described in the previous chapters accomplish this in an efficient and effective manner.

When cases present with high mandibular plane angles, extraction treatment is considered (673). High angle cases with minimal crowding, minimal protrusion of incisors, and sufficient anterior overbite can be treated on a non-extraction basis. When high angle cases show protrusion and/or crowding of incisors with minimal overbite or open bite tendencies, then extractions are necessary.

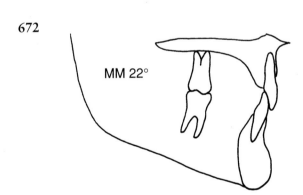

MM 22°

672 In general, when cases present with average to low mandibular plane angles, every attempt is made to treat on a non-extraction basis. However, when low angle cases show excessive protrusion and/or crowding, extraction treatment must be carried out.

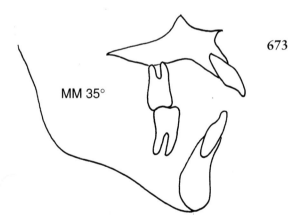

MM 35°

673 When cases present with high mandibular plane angles, extraction treatment is considered.

674

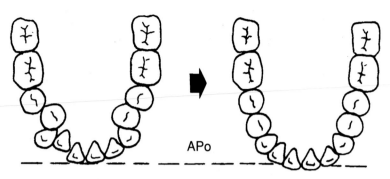

A major challenge of non-extraction treatment is the gaining of adequate space in the arches to provide a stable end-result. There are four primary methods in which space can be gained in the non-extraction case:

- Advancement of incisors (674).
- Uprighting of molars (675).
- Lateral expansion (676).
- Interproximal stripping (677).

674 Advancement of incisors. For each mm of mesial movement of lower incisors, 2 mm of space is gained (1 mm per side).

675

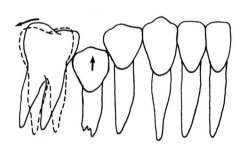

676

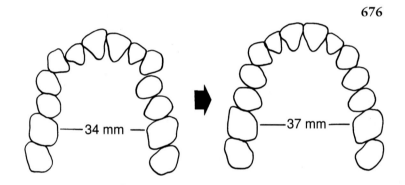

675 Uprighting of molars. When necessary, lower molars can be uprighted by approximately 1 mm per side in most cases, providing a total of 2 mm of additional space.

676 Lateral expansion. While there are limits to arch expansion due to available alveolar bone, it is often possible to gain space with expansion procedures.

677

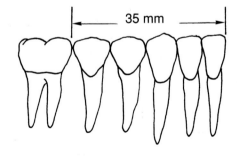

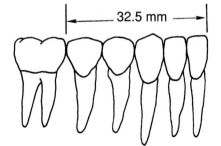

677 Interproximal enamel reduction can be effectively utilized to gain space in the upper and lower arches and to co-ordinate tooth sizes in the arches.

Advancement of Incisors

For each millimeter of mesial movement of the lower incisors, 2 mm of space is gained (1 mm per side). Lower incisors can be safely advanced by 2 mm in many cases, for example, to give a total gain of 4 mm of space (674). A discussion of lower incisor advancement was presented in Chapter 9. In Class I results, the authors prefer lower incisors to be positioned approximately 2 mm in front of APo and at 95° to the mandibular plane.

However, rigid adherence to cephalometric normals is often not in the patient's best interest. For example, when treating a Class I case with slight crowding on a non-extraction basis, if lower incisors must be left at APo +3.5 mm, this can be an acceptable compromise. The alternative in such a case would be to extract first bicuspids, which is often not warranted when lower incisors can be left 1.5 mm forward of the average or normal.

Dental compensation from an ideal lower incisor position may be required in Class III and Class II skeletal cases. In Class III cases, compensation is often necessary to keep the lower incisors in a more upright position (for example APo 0) and upper incisors in a more forward position. This is necessary to compensate for the skeletal Class III pattern (678).

In Class II cases compensation is often necessary to leave lower incisors in a more forward position (for example APo + 4) with the upper incisors in a more upright position, to compensate for the Class II skeletal pattern. This can reduce the need to over-retract the maxillary incisors, and thus avoid flattening of the facial profile (679). In this compensatory situation, there may be a tendency for post-orthodontic incisor crowding, but this can be dealt with in the retention phase of treatment and is an acceptable compromise.

ANB 1°

678

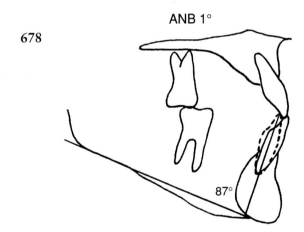

87°

ANB 5°

679

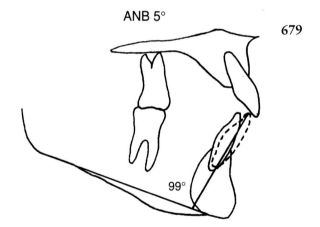

99°

678 In Class III skeletal cases it is often necessary to leave the lower incisors in a more retroclined position, to compensate for the dental base discrepancy.

679 In Class II skeletal cases it is often necessary to leave the lower incisors in a more proclined position, to compensate for the dental base discrepancy.

Uprighting or Distalizing of Molars

Upper molars can be distalized 2–4 mm when necessary to provide additional space in the upper arch. The methods of distalization of the upper first molars were discussed in detail in Chapter 9 and they include:

- Facebow headgears
- Class II elastics to upper sliding jigs
- Class II elastics to the entire upper arch

When necessary, lower molars can be uprighted by approximately 1 mm per side in most cases, providing a total of 2 mm of additional space. This can be achieved with the following procedures:

- Tip-back bends in the lower archwire
- Lip bumpers
- Open coil springs
- Reverse sliding jigs to the lower arch
- Class III elastics to the entire lower arch

Tip-back bends in the lower archwire

While the normal archform used during treatment does not involve the placement of second order bends in the posterior segments, there are situations when such bends are advantageous. When lower molars are tipped forward, the use of tip-back bends is helpful in the uprighting process. These bends can be supplemented with open coil springs and Class III elastics.

Lip bumpers

Lower molar brackets can be provided with extra tubes into which a lip bumper can be placed for purposes of uprighting the lower molars, as shown in Chapter 4. The lip bumper is designed to extend approximately 2 mm in front of the lower incisors at the gingival aspect of these teeth. Hooks can also be soldered to the lip bumper in the anterior region so that Class III elastics can be attached from upper first molars to these hooks, greatly accelerating the uprighting process. When Class III elastics are used, it is normally advantageous to fit a palatal bar and headgear to the upper arch, to stabilize upper first molar positions.

Open coil springs

When there is loss of space in the lower arch due to premature loss of deciduous molars, an open coil spring can be placed mesial to the first molars for uprighting purposes. If the space loss is unilateral, it may also be helpful to place a lower lingual arch from the first molar on one side to the first bicuspid on the other side, for stabilization (**680**).

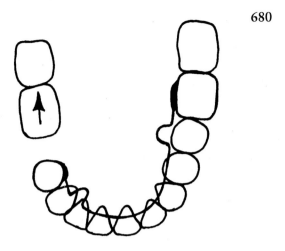

680

680 If the space loss is unilateral, it may be advantageous to place a lower lingual arch from the first molar on one side of the arch to the first bicuspid on the other side, for stabilization.

Reverse sliding jigs to the lower arch

In cases with severely tipped first molars, a sliding jig can be placed mesial to these molars and Class III elastics used for uprighting. This is effective on one or both sides of the arch.

Palatal bars and headgears should also be considered for stabilization of upper first molars whenever Class III elastics are employed to support anchorage in the lower arch.

Class III elastics

Class III elastics can be carried to the entire lower arch for the purposes of uprighting and distalization of the lower molars.

Arch Expansion

It is often possible to gain space by expansion procedures within certain limits, depending on the amount of available alveolar bone. There are three methods to create space in this lateral direction when necessary:

- Expansion of the mid-palatal suture in the upper arch — RME (681–86).
- Buccal uprighting of teeth in the upper and lower arches.
- Dento-alveolar expansion in the upper and lower arches.

Expansion of the mid-palatal suture

The technique of rapid maxillary expansion has proved effective in creating space in the upper arch (681). This expansion may be considered until the late teens or early twenties when fusion of the mid-palatal suture occurs.[1] The palatal expander is normally attached to bands on the first molars and first bicuspids (683). Initially, this appliance is activated one quarter turn per day, providing .25 mm of expansion. Once the mid-palatal suture begins to separate and the patient is comfortable with the appliance, activation can occur twice a day, providing .50 mm of expansion (682–686).

When adequate expansion has been achieved, the appliance can be stabilized with a ligature wire and left in place for three months, while bone is deposited in the mid-palatal suture area. Alternatively, the rapid expansion appliance can be replaced by a simple palatal arch for stabilization, while bony reorganization occurs.

681

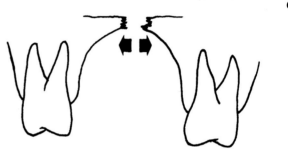

681 The technique of rapid maxillary expansion has proved effective in creating space in the upper arch.

Buccal uprighting

Buccal uprighting of posterior segments is the normal method of expansion that occurs in the lower arch and frequently can be carried out in combination with mid-palatal suture expansion in the upper arch.

It is important to note that the archform used by the authors, and shown in Chapter 2, has proved effective in achieving buccal uprighting in the bicuspid regions. This archform has been used for more than ten years and it pro-vides proper positioning of the bicuspids so that during protrusive functional movements, the lower bicuspids can make contact with the upper cuspids.

Thus, while the archform is slightly wider in the bicuspid region than the arches of most patients, an acceptable adaptation seems to occur between the tongue lingually and the cheeks buccally, allowing for a stable end position of the involved teeth.

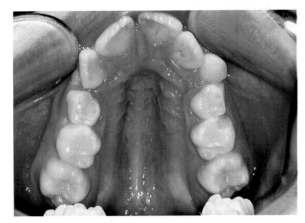

682 A narrow maxilla in a Class III case with low tongue position.

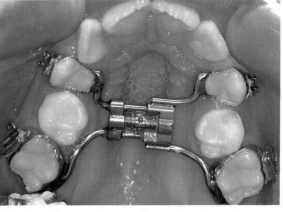

683 Rapid expansion appliance in place after completion of 28 turns.

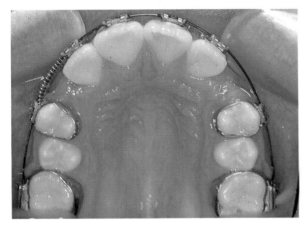

684 Progressive placement of fixed appliances, with a coil spring active 1 mm to re-create space for the upper right canine.

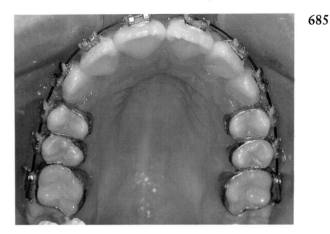

685 Completion of preliminary leveling and aligning, using slightly expanded archwires.

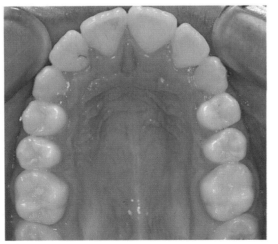

686 The upper arch at the end of treatment, with canines in alignment. Often the tongue adopts an improved posture when archform is re-established in this way.

Dento-alveolar expansion

It is possible to create a limited amount of space with dento-alveolar expansion using slightly expanded archforms. Each case must be evaluated prior to treatment to determine if there is adequate bone for this type of expansion. For example, in cases where there is tapering of the buccal bone in the maxilla, above the dentition, it is unlikely that space can be gained by dento-alveolar expansion.

However, if the buccal alveolar processes are broad, 1 or 2 mm of expansion per side can be attempted and often achieved.

Interproximal Stripping

Interproximal enamel stripping can be effectively used to gain space in the upper and lower arches and also to co-ordinate tooth sizes between the two arches (see **702–704**).

Since each tooth has .75 to 1.25 mm of interproximal enamel on each surface, it is safe to remove .25 mm of enamel from the contact areas of these teeth. This removal reduces the space between each root by approximately .50 mm and there is no evidence that this reduction creates periodontal disadvantages or an increased risk of tooth decay, provided oral hygiene is reasonably good. From the mesial of the first molar on one side of the arch to the mesial of the first molar on the opposite side of the arch, there are 22 tooth surfaces. If .25 mm of enamel is removed from each of these surfaces, a total of 5.5 mm of space can be gained. Enamel reduction is only carried out when necessary. If it means the difference between extraction and non-extraction treatment, particularly in an average to low angle case, then the procedure is acceptable.

Summary

The authors make every attempt to treat their cases on a non-extraction basis. This chapter has described the most effective methods of gaining space to avoid extractions.

However, if it is felt that non-extraction treatment will create an unstable, periodontally compromised, unesthetic or unacceptable functional end-result, such as a result with an open bite and molar fulcruming, then extractions must be considered. This book is dedicated to helping the orthodontist to avoid the pitfalls of extraction treatment. These include unacceptable flattening of the facial profile, tipping of teeth into extraction sites, open extraction sites, and bite deepening.

CASE REPORT JT

A Class I non-extraction case

A 13-year-old boy with a Class I skeletal and dental pattern, showing moderate protrusion of his upper and lower incisors. There was slight to moderate crowding in his upper and lower anterior segments.

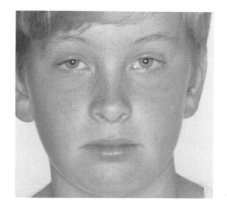

687

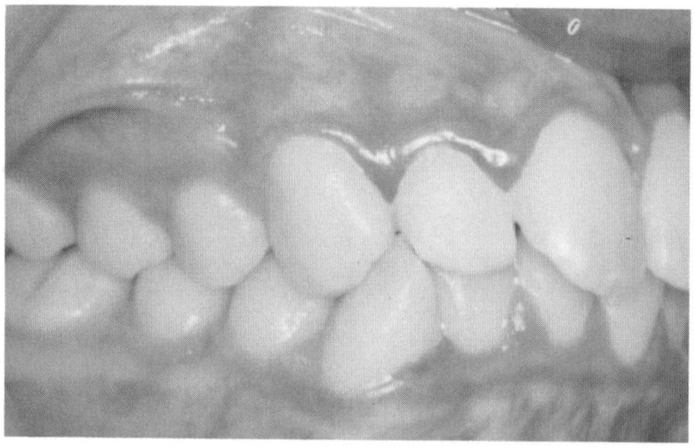

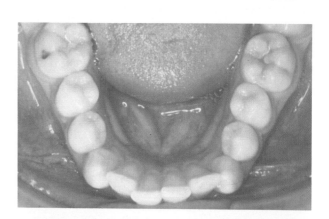

690

A decision was made to treat on a non-extraction basis, with interproximal stripping.

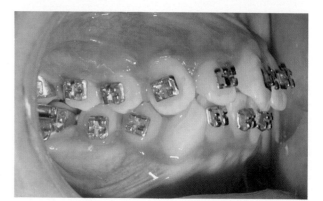

693

All teeth were banded or bracketed, except for the second molars and the lower canines.

696

688

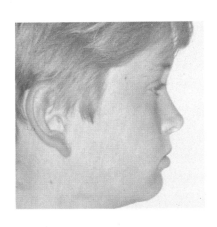

689

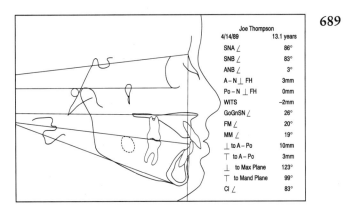

Joe Thompson
4/14/89   13.1 years

SNA ∠	86°
SNB ∠	83°
ANB ∠	3°
A – N ⊥ FH	3mm
Po – N ⊥ FH	0mm
WITS	–2mm
GoGnSN ∠	26°
FM ∠	20°
MM ∠	19°
⊥ to A – Po	10mm
⊤ to A – Po	3mm
⊥ to Max Plane	123°
⊤ to Mand Plane	99°
CI ∠	83°

691

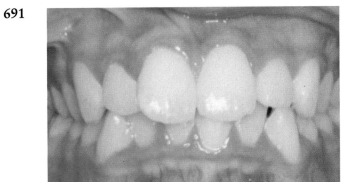

692

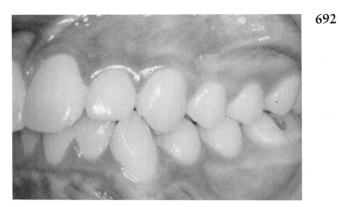

694

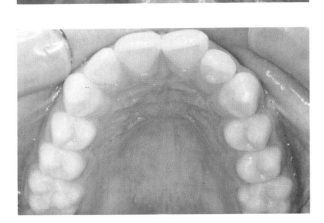

695

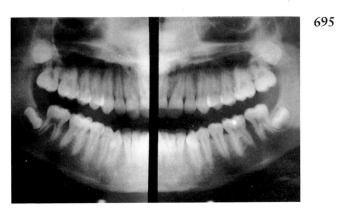

697

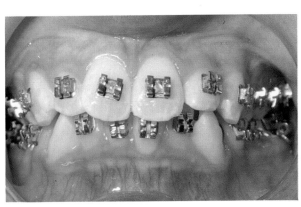

698

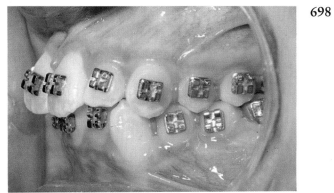

The sequence of interproximal stripping was as follows:

- Visit 1 — stripping of the mesial of the first molars and the distal of the second premolars.
- Visit 2 — stripping of the mesial of the second premolars, the mesial and distal of the first premolars, and the distal of the canines.
- Visit 3 — stripping of the mesial surface of the canines, the mesial and distal surface of the lateral incisors, and the distal surface of the central incisors.

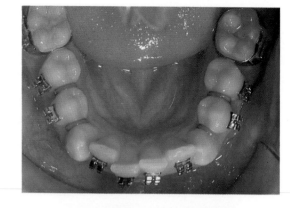

699

The extent of interproximal stripping was .25 mm per contact area which provided approximately 5 mm of space in each of the upper and lower arches. A high-speed handpiece was used with a Brasseler ET-3 diamond burr under water spray.

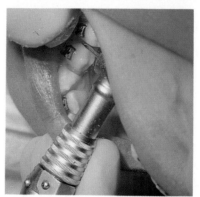

702

An upper headgear and a lower lip bumper were used to maintain molar position, and the upper canines were retracted using lacebacks.

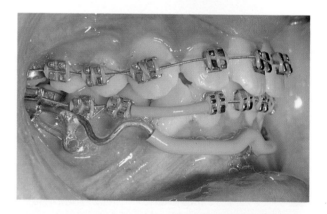

705

Coil springs were used, with 1 mm of activation, to increase the space for the lower canines.

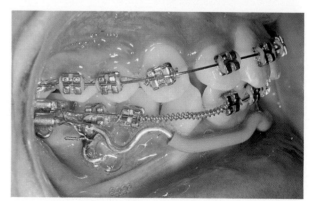

708

700

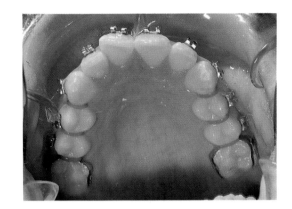

701

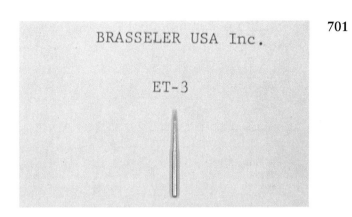

703

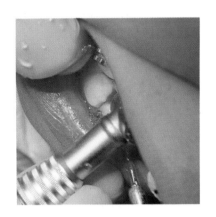

704

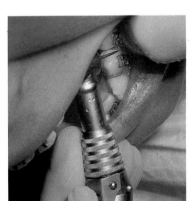

706

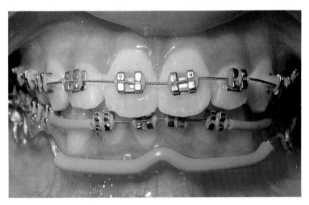

707

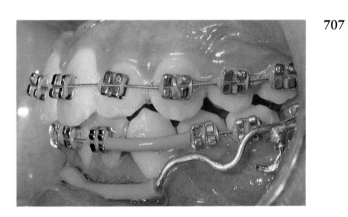

709

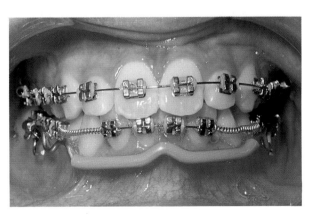

710

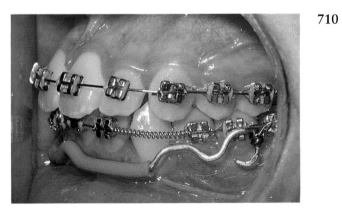

After three months of treatment, brackets were bonded onto the lower canines.

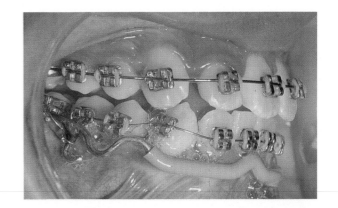

711

Rotation wedges were used to rotate the lower canines, and active tiebacks were used in the upper arch, with a .019/.025 rectangular wire. The case is five months into treatment.

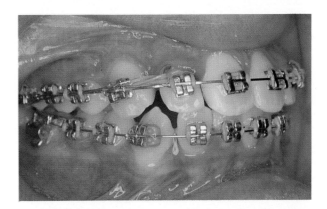

714

Upper space has almost closed and lower leveling and aligning is continuing, after six months of treatment.

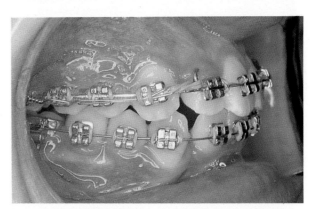

717

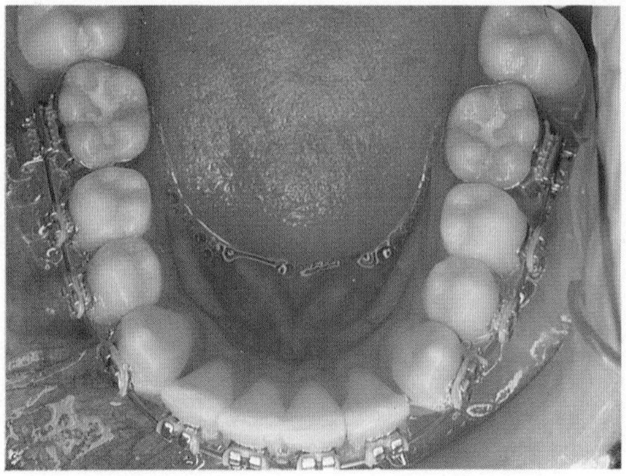

720

712 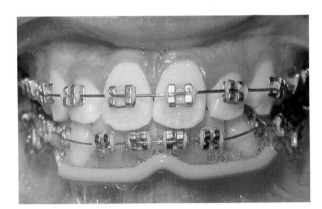 713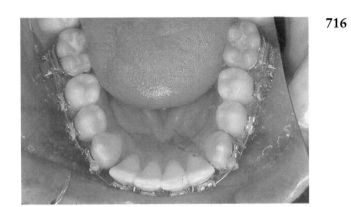

715 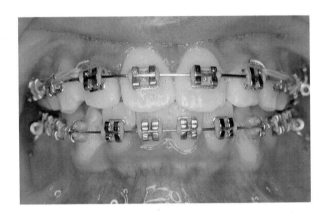 716

718 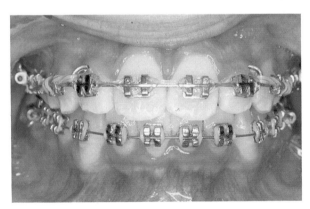 719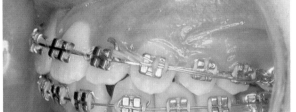

721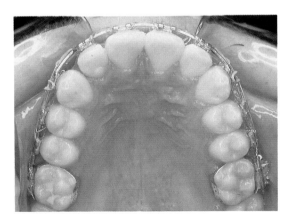

After one year of treatment, with upper and lower rectangular wires in place, and passive tiebacks to prevent spaces from opening.

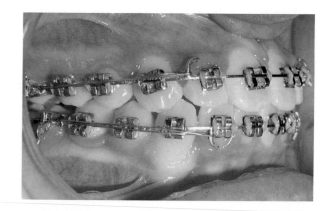

722

Progressive band removal was carried out, after 15 months of active treatment.

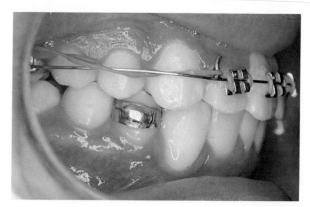

725

An upper removable Hawley retainer was worn at night. A fixed lower premolar-to-premolar retainer was cemented in place.

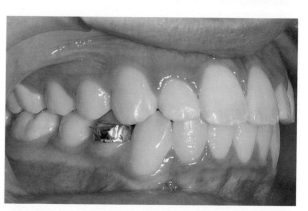

728

The lower incisors were maintained in their original position and the upper incisors were retracted by approximately 2 mm.

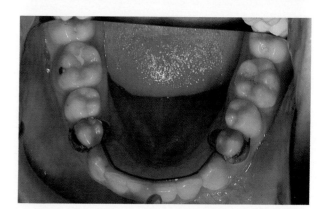

731

723
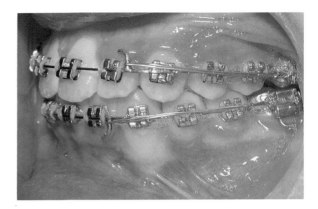
724

726
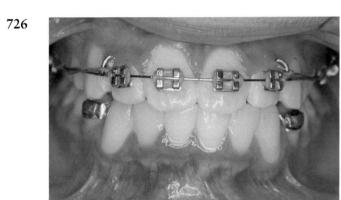
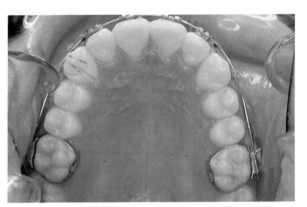
727

729
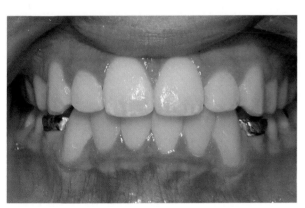
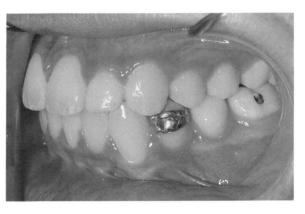
730

732
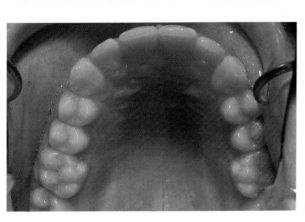
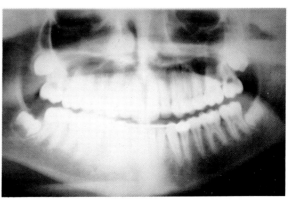
733

734

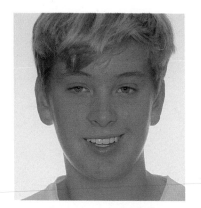

735

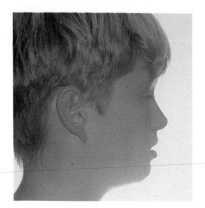

736

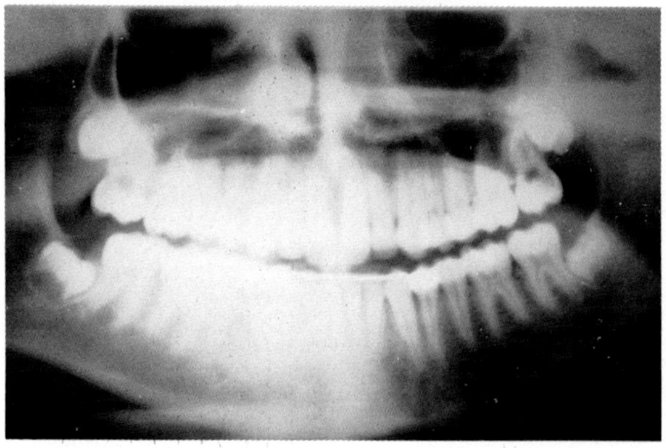

737

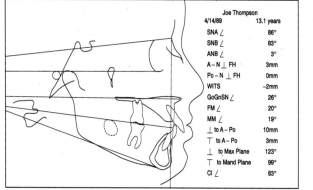

Joe Thompson

4/14/89	13.1 years
SNA ∠	86°
SNB ∠	83°
ANB ∠	3°
A – N ⊥ FH	3mm
Po – N ⊥ FH	0mm
WITS	–2mm
GoGnSN ∠	26°
FM ∠	20°
MM ∠	19°
⊥ to A – Po	10mm
⊤ to A – Po	3mm
⊥ to Max Plane	123°
⊤ to Mand Plane	99°
CI ∠	83°

738

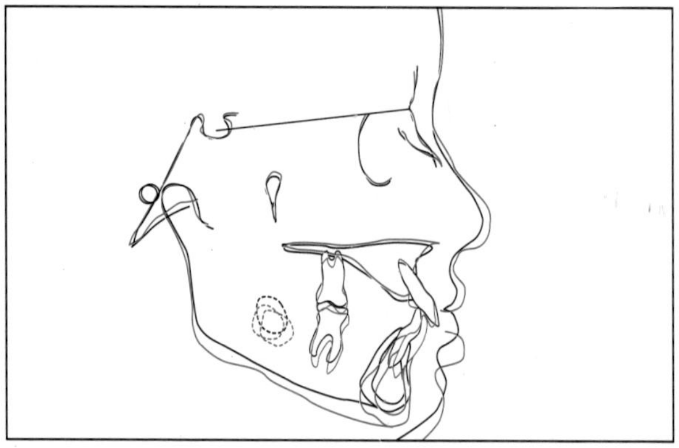

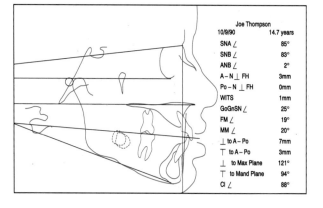

739

Joe Thompson

10/9/90	14.7 years
SNA ∠	85°
SNB ∠	83°
ANB ∠	2°
A – N ⊥ FH	3mm
Po – N ⊥ FH	0mm
WITS	1mm
GoGnSN ∠	25°
FM ∠	19°
MM ∠	20°
⊥ to A – Po	7mm
⊤ to A – Po	3mm
⊥ to Max Plane	121°
⊤ to Mand Plane	94°
CI ∠	88°

CASE REPORT WD

A Class II malocclusion showing space gaining
by molar uprighting, advancement of incisors,
and slight expansion.

A boy aged 11 years and 11 months showing a slight Class II skeletal and dental pattern. There was a deep overbite, a short lower face height, and significant crowding in upper and lower arches.

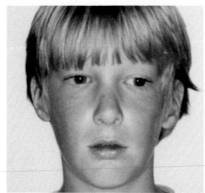

740

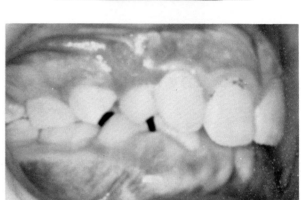

743

Occlusal views confirm the lack of space in this moderately crowded case.

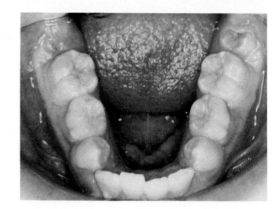

746

741

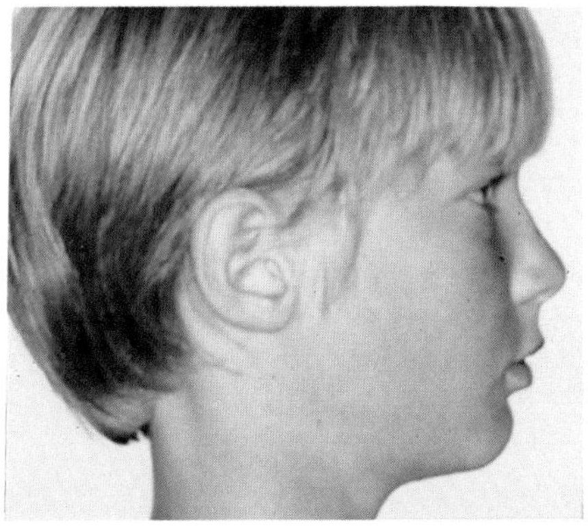

742

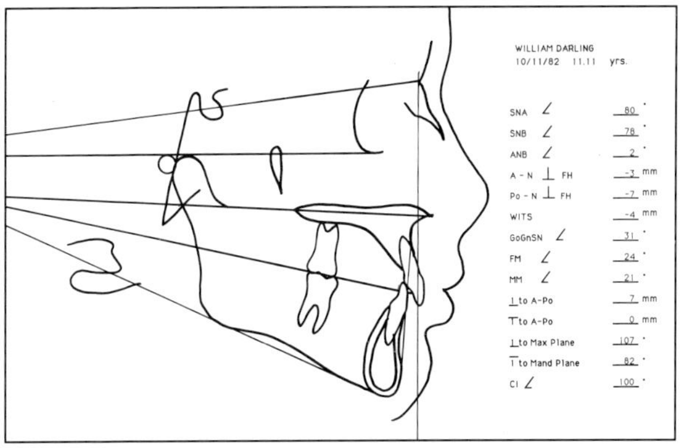

WILLIAM DARLING
10/11/82 11.11 yrs.

SNA ∠	80	°
SNB ∠	78	°
ANB ∠	2	°
A - N ⊥ FH	-3	mm
Po - N ⊥ FH	-7	mm
WITS	-4	mm
GoGnSN ∠	31	°
FM ∠	24	°
MM ∠	21	°
⊥ to A-Po	7	mm
⊤ to A-Po	0	mm
⊥ to Max Plane	107	°
⊤ to Mand Plane	82	°
CI ∠	100	°

744

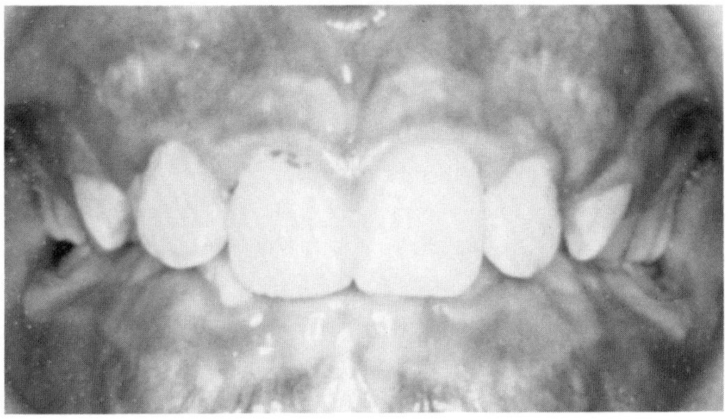

745

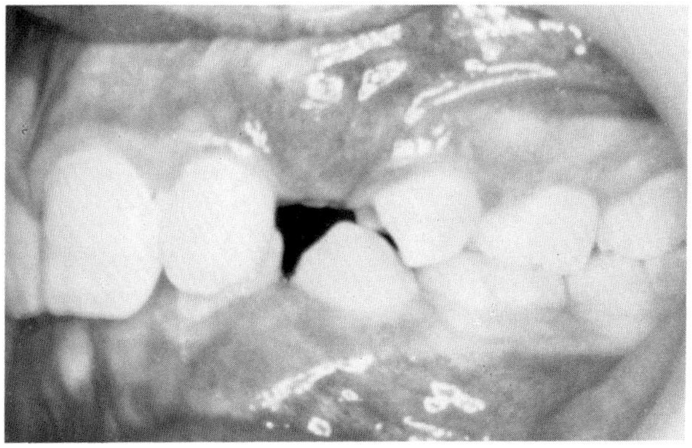

747

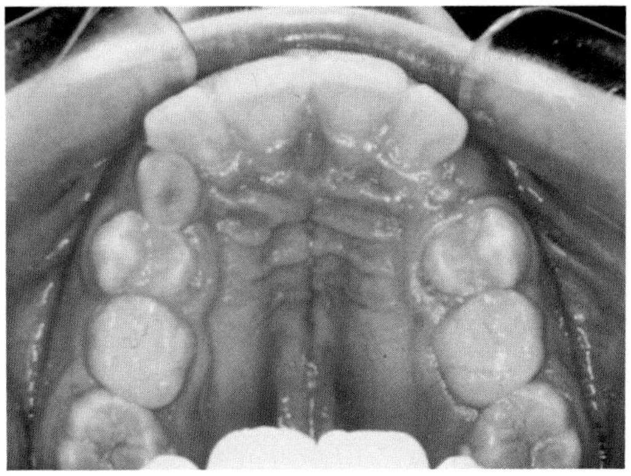

748

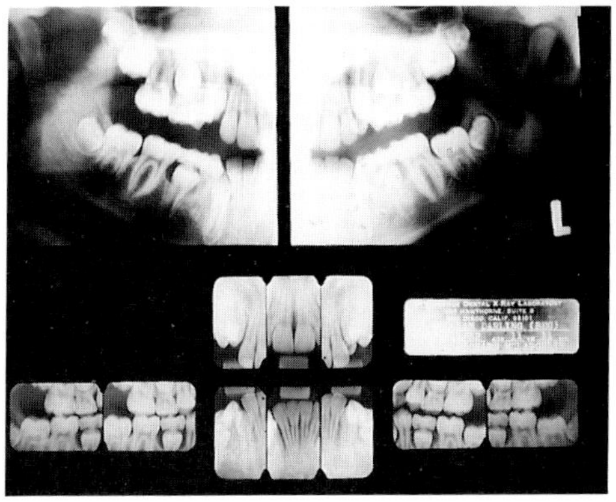

The patient was treated on a non-extraction basis, using a lower utility arch to intrude incisors and tip back the molars. The patient was asked to wear a headgear at night to distalize the upper molars.

749

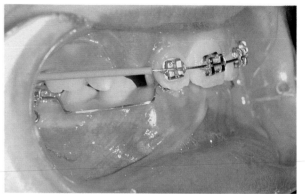

752

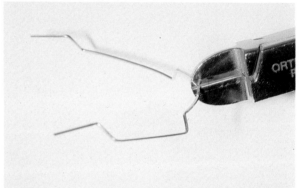

Soft elastic sleeving was used for patient comfort, and to protect the archwire.

755

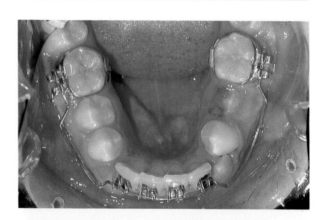

Lower molars uprighting in response to the archwire which was designed as shown in **752–754**.

758

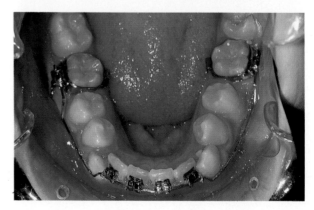

750
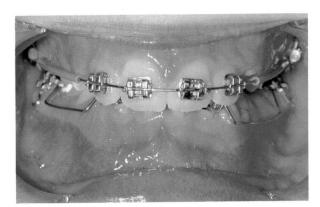

751
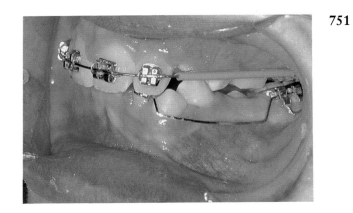

753
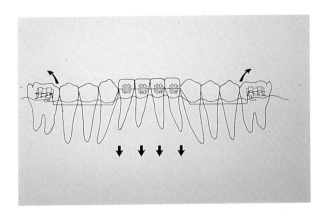

754
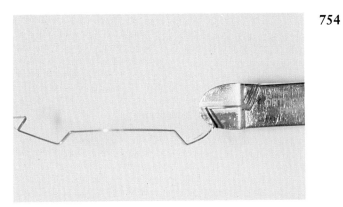

756
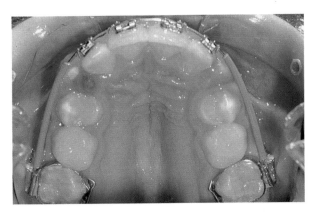

757
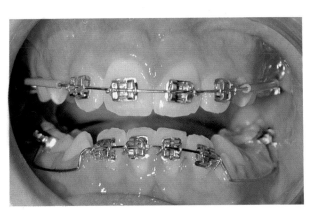

759
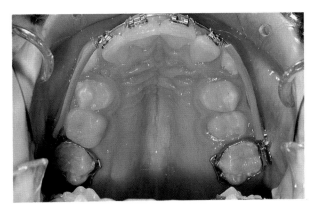

When the lower incisors had been intruded, and the molars uprighted, upper and lower arches were fully banded for routine levelling and aligning. This resulted in slight advancement of the incisors and slight expansion of the arches.

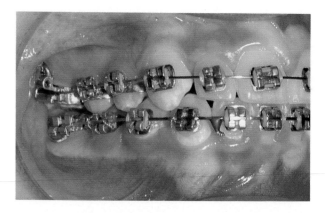

760

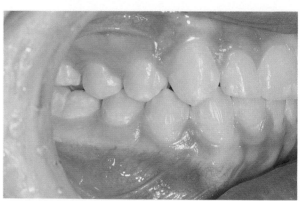

763

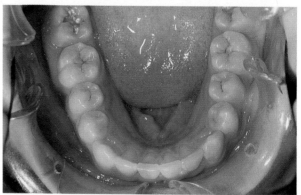

766

Final records show that the incisors were advanced approximately 2–3mm.

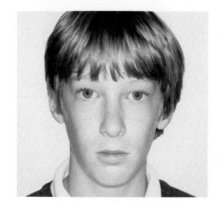

769

761

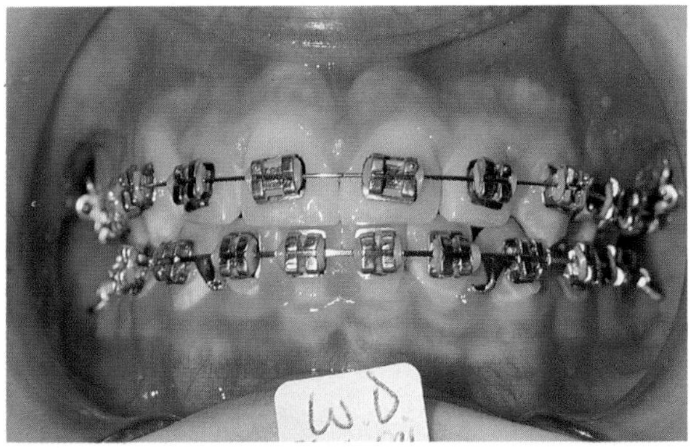

762

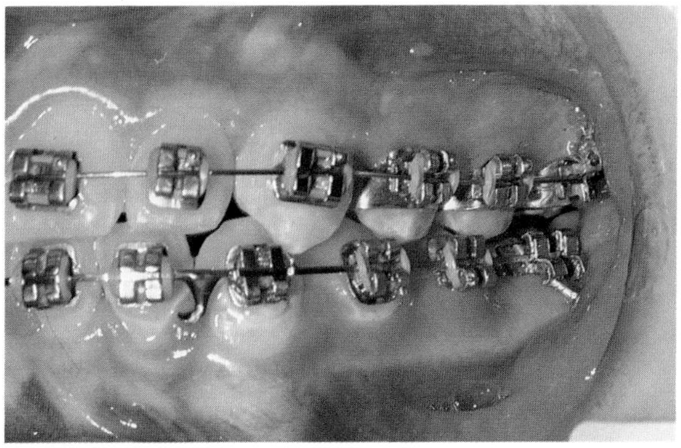

764

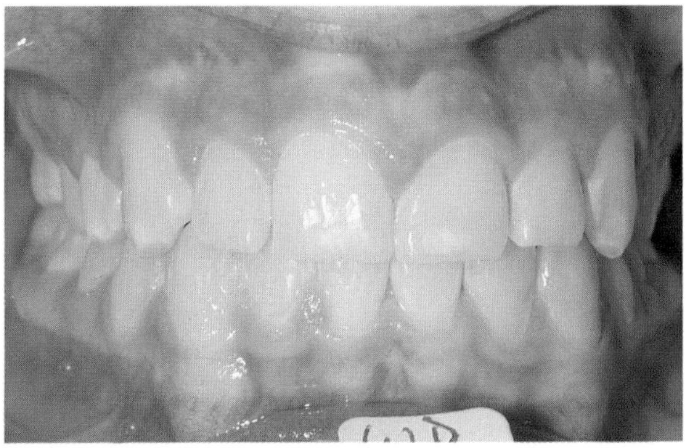

765

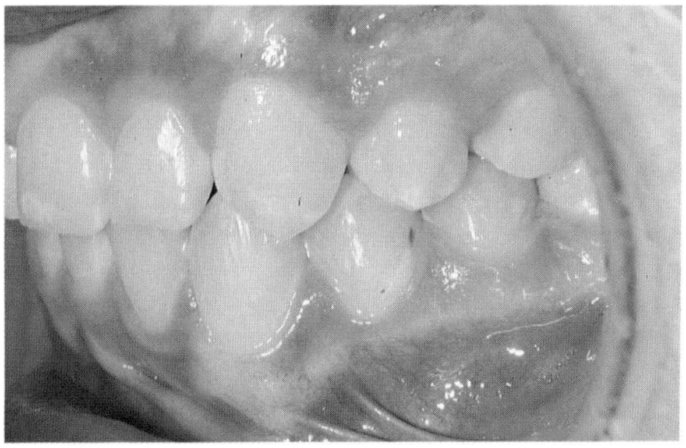

767

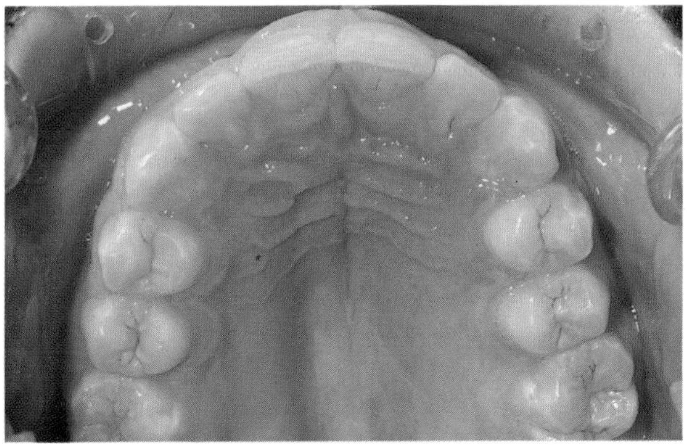

768

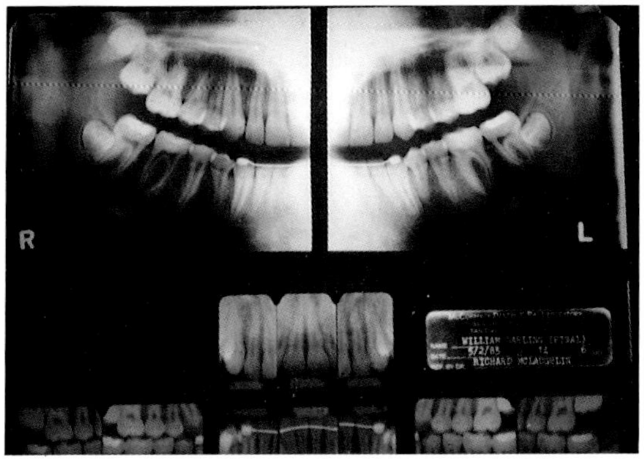

770

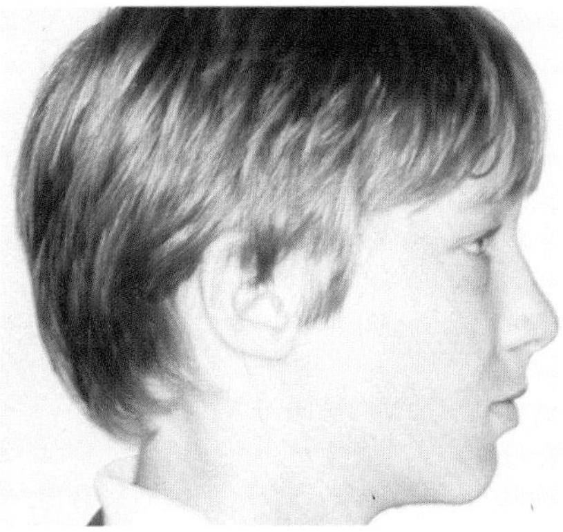

771

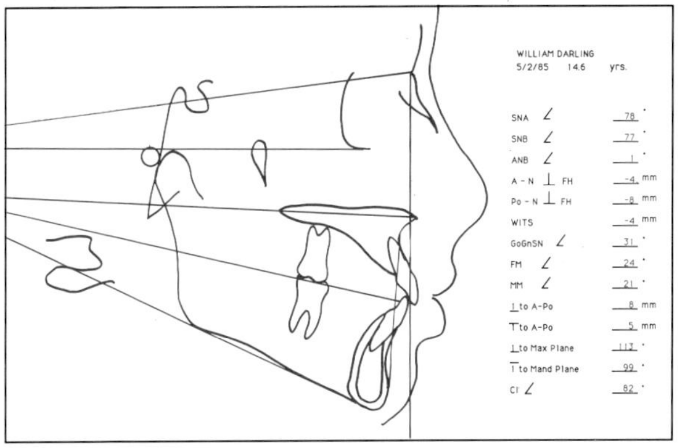

WILLIAM DARLING	
5/2/85 14.6 yrs.	
SNA ∠	78 °
SNB ∠	77 °
ANB ∠	1 °
A - N ⊥ FH	-4 mm
Po - N ⊥ FH	-8 mm
WITS	-4 mm
GoGnSN ∠	31 °
FM ∠	24 °
MM ∠	21 °
1 to A-Po	8 mm
⊤ to A-Po	5 mm
1 to Max Plane	117 °
⊤ to Mand Plane	99 °
CI ∠	82 °

Records taken four years later show that the case is stable, following treatment which included a small amount of expansion and advancement of incisors.

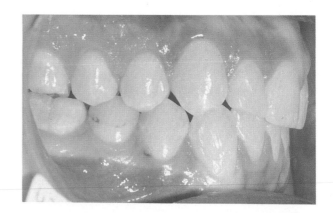

772

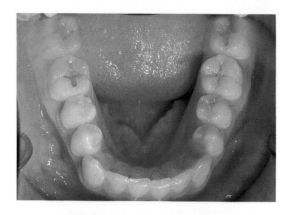

775

By treating on a non-extraction basis, it was possible to achieve a very satisfactory result for this low angle case. If teeth had been extracted, it is likely that the patient would have had an unacceptably flat facial profile.

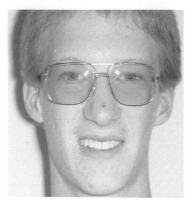

777

773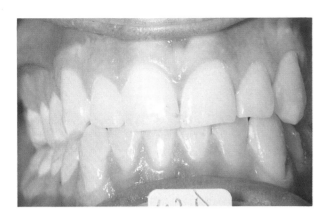

774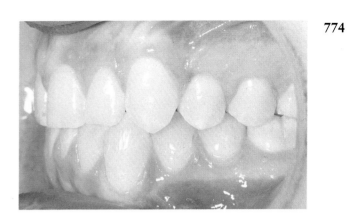

776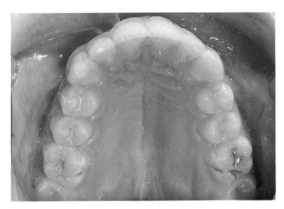

778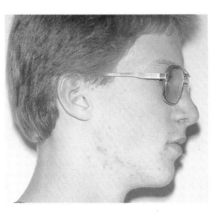

779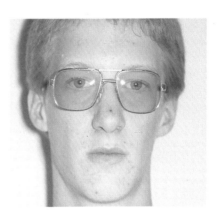

REFERENCES

3. Appliance Selection

1. McLaughlin, R.P. and Bennett J.C., 'The Transition from Standard Edgewise to Preadjusted Appliance Systems', *J. Clin. Orth.* **23**: 142–153, 1989.
2. *The 'A' Company Straight-Wire Appliance.* An eight page descriptive brochure published by 'A' Co., San Diego, CA, USA, a Johnson & Johnson Company.
3. Andrews, L.F., 'The Six Keys to Normal Occlusion', *Am. J. Orth.* **62**: 296–309, 1972.

4. Appliance Variations

1. Andrews, L.F., *Straight-Wire — The Concept and The Appliance*, L.A. Wells Co., 1989.

6. The Transition from Standard Edgewise to Preadjusted Appliance Systems

1. Holdaway, R.A. 'Bracket Angulation as Applied to the Edgewise Appliance, *Angle Orthodontist,* **22**: 227, 1952.
2. Andrews, L.F., 'The Six Keys to Normal Occlusion', *Am. J. Orth.* **62**: 296–309, 1972.
3. 'JCO Study of Orthodontic Diagnosis and Treatment Procedures', *J. Clin Orth.,* **20**: 573, 1986.
4. Andrews, L.F., Advanced II Straight-Wire Appliance Course, Dec. 1–3, 1979..
5. Tweed, C.H., *Clinical Orthodontics*, St Louis: C.V. Mosby, 1966.
6. Andrews, L.F., *The Straight-Wire Appliance — Syllabus of Philosophy and Technique,* 2nd Ed., 1975.
7. Roth, R.H., 'The Straight-Wire Appliance 17 Years Later', *J. Clin. Orth.* **21**: 632–642, 1987.

7. Anchorage Control during Leveling and Aligning

1. Andrews, L.F., *The Straight-Wire Appliance: Syllabus of Philosophy and Technique,* 2nd Ed., 1975.
2. Roth, R.H., 'The Straight-Wire Appliance 17 Years Later', *J. Clin. Orth.* **21**: 632–642, 1987.
3. Robinson, S.N., 'An evaluation of the changes in lower incisor position during the initial stages of clinical treatment using a preadjusted edgewise appliance', MSc Thesis, Univ. of London, 1989.

8. The Management of Increased Overbite

1. McLaughlin, R.P. and Bennett J.C., 'The Transition from Standard Edgewise to Preadjusted Appliance Systems', *J. Clin. Orth.* **23**: 142–153, 1989.
2. Bennett, J.C. and McLaughlin R.P., 'Controlled Space Closure with a Preadjusted Appliance System', *J. Clin. Orth.* **24**: 251–260, 1990.
3. Steiner, C., 'Cephalometrics for You and Me', *Am. J. Orth.* **39**: 729–755, 1953.
4. Riolo, M. et al, *An Atlas of Craniofacial Growth*, Center for Human Growth and Development, Univ. of Michigan, 1974.

9. Overjet Reduction

1. Riolo, M. et al, *An Atlas of Craniofacial Growth*, Center for Human Growth and Development, Univ. of Michigan, 1974.
2. Steiner, C., 'Cephalometrics for You and Me', *Am. J. Orth.* **39**: 729–755, 1953.
3. McNamara, J.A., 'A Method of Cephalometric Evaluation', *Am. J. Orth.* **86**: 449–469, 1984.
4. Jacobson, A., 'The "Wits" Appraisal of Jaw Disharmony', *Am. J. Orth.* **67**: 138–155, 1975.
5. Moyers, R.E., 'Differential Diagnosis of Class II Malocclusions', *Am. J. Orth.* **78**: 477–494, 1980.
6. Bjork, A., 'Mandibular Growth Rotation', *J. Dental Research* **42**: 400–411, 1963.
7. Harvold, E.P., *The Activator in Interceptive Orthodontics*, C.V. Mosby, St Louis, 1974.
8. Mills, J.R.E., 'Clinical Control of Craniofacial Growth: A Skeptic's Viewpoint', in: McNamara, J.A. and Ribbens K.A., (Eds.) *Face, Craniofacial Growth Series*, Monograph No. 14, Univ. of Michigan, pp. 17–39, 1983.
9. Graber, 'Heavy Intermittent Cervical Traction in Class II Treatment: A Longitudinal Cephalometric Asessment', *Am. J. Orth.* **74**: 361–387, 1978.
10. Andrews, L.F., *The Straight-Wire Appliance: Syllabus of Philosophy and Technique,* 2nd Ed., 1975.

10. Space Closure Procedures

1. Andrews, L.F., *The Straight Wire Appliance: Syllabus of Philosophy and Technique,* 2nd Ed., 1975.
2. Gottleib, E.L.; Nelson, A.H. and Vogels, D.S., 'JCO Study of Orth. Diag. and Treatment Procedures', *J. Clin. Orth.* **20**: 612-625, 1986.
3. Rudge, S.J., personal communication.
4. Muira F., Mogi M., Ohura Y., Karibe, M., 'The Superelastic Japanese Ni Ti alloy wire for use in Orthodontics. Part 3. Studies on the Japanese Ni Ti alloy coil springs', *Am. J. Orth.* **94**: 89-96, 1988.
5. Bennett, J.C. and McLaughlin R.P. 'Controlled Space Closure with a Preadjusted Appliance System', *J. Clin. Orth.* **24**: 251-260, 1990.

11. Finishing and Detailing

1. Dougherty, H.L., Lecture series on finishing and detailing, University of Southern California, April 1976.
2. Andrews, L.F., 'The Straight Wire Appliance Explained and Compared', *J. Clin. Orth.* **10**: 174–195, 1976.
3. Roth, R., 'Gnathological Concepts and Orthodontic Treatment Goals', in Jarabak J.R. and Fizzell J.A. (Eds.), *Technique and Treatment with Light Wire Appliances,* 2nd. Ed., C.V. Mosby, pp. 1160–1223, 1972.
4. McLaughlin, R.P. and Bennett J. C., 'Finishing and Detailing with a Preadjusted Appliance System', *J. Clin. Orth.* **25**: 251-264, 1991.

12. Non-extraction Treatment

1. Timms, D.J., *Rapid Maxillary Expansion,* Quintessence Publishing Co., Inc., 1981.

INDEX

Location references are page numbers.